Praise for *Eat Rec*

"Nicolette is like an encouraging best friend who takes you by the hand and leads you into a new way of eating and living. She's not preaching a gimmicky weight loss diet or a 'miracle' powder or pill. She's preaching about real, unprocessed food that's packed with nutrients—food that makes your body say, 'Thank you. This feels so good!' Keep this book in your kitchen and it will serve as a daily reminder to take excellent care of your body—after all, it's the only one you've got!"

—**Alexandra Franzen**, author of *You're Going to Survive*

"What a wonderful read! Nicolette describes in detail the specific protocols for implementing the Gerson Therapy, but she also offers us a plethora of tools in setting ourselves up for optimum health success."

—**Nancy Kremer**, writer/producer, *Dr. Max Gerson: Healing the Hopeless* feature film

"Richer smoothly guides us through an attainable step by step healing process. She alleviates the daunting and overwhelming fears around overcoming illness with a simple and necessary tool to heal, giving those traumatized with a negative diagnosis a real chance at living again."

—**Erica Nasby**, Personal Development Coach and Speaker, Exit Reality Corp.

"Nicolette Richer not only makes the science of healing and long-term health easy to understand, she breaks it down into very consumable chunks (no pun intended). I have known her for many years and I trust her advice completely. Every bit of what she recommends has been thoroughly researched and tested on herself and her family. This is not a fad diet. This is for real! And it works. I recommend this book to anyone who wants to live a long and healthful life."

—**Sylvia Dolson**, author, aspiring centenarian, and animal welfare advocate

"Working alongside [Nicolette] and watching this project, and the beautiful 'PS I Love You' campaign, come to life was nothing short of incredible. So many people reach out to her for help. In writing this book she will be able to reach all of them, creating a ripple effect that will touch many lives forever."

—**Stephie Hennekam**, Certified Dietitian, plant-based yogi and Richer Health team player

"Eat real food. Be healthy. Nicolette shares a simple, powerful idea with us all in this wonderful book. Her heartfelt message is backed up by years of experience, and a solid plan on how to live and eat well. This book condenses Nicolette's wonderful advice into a convenient package to keep at home. You can hear her voice in every page, full of enthusiasm and joy at sharing the simple, beautiful idea of eating real to heal. Try it. Feel it. Believe it."

—**Selene Moore**, teacher, artist, mom and Eat Real to Heal convert

"It would be hard to find a more energetic, enthusiastic proponent of natural health than Nicolette Richer.... This book is more than just a dietary recommendation. It is vastly more than that, including sections on exercise, meditation, parenting, and healing, all with good humor and wry wit, and a love of humanity, family and friends that is rare to see in these contentious times."

—**Howard Straus**

EAT
REAL
to
HEAL

Eat Real to Heal: Using Nutrient Dense Foods for Longevity and Happiness

This book is not intended as a substitute for the medical advice of
physicians. The reader should regularly consult a physician in matters
relating to his or her health and particularly with respect to any symptoms
that may require diagnosis or medical attention.

ISBN: (print) 978-1-68481-416-9 (ebook) 978-1-68481-472-5
Library of Congress Control Number: 2018952296
BISAC category code: CKB103000, COOKING / Health & Healing / Cancer

Dr. Nicolette Richer's

EAT
REAL
to
HEAL

Using Nutrient Dense Foods for Longevity and Happiness

CORAL GABLES

ps: i love you

-Eat Real to Heal-

Dear

PS: I love you,

EAT REAL
TO HEAL

www.eatrealtoheal.ca

ps: i love you

-Eat Real to Heal-

What is our 'PS: I Love You' campaign about?

It's a campaign that flowed from my book 'Eat Real to Heal'. The book is inspired by my own Gerson journey and my mission to teach the world how to eat and beat any disease.

It is perfect for those who are looking to (re)connect with loved one(s) and get on the healing train together. The book has tons of recipes, inspiring healing stories, worksheets to keep your progress rolling and more.

It's a campaign where instead of telling someone who is battling a chronic illness or cancer to do this or do that, read this, watch that, or (don't) eat this... You simply tell them: PS: I Love You!

But more importantly, PS I love you is an invitation to explore, research and adopt a plant-based, whole food lifestyle because... I love you. I want you to be healthy, vibrant, disease free and have energy. I want to live a joyful life with you for as long as possible!

PS also means Plant Strong. Plant strong means you choose veggies over processed foods, you choose fruits and grains over packaged fake food. Plant strong means your body is thriving and is loving you and rewarding you for it.

I love you means... I love you.

www.eatrealtoheal.ca

Contents

FOREWORD

I am delighted to pen down these words as a foreword to a book that will change your life, transform your perspective, and revolutionize how you approach your health. I've been around in the health and fitness world for over twenty years, and let me tell you, this is a game-changer. *Eat Real to Heal* by Dr. Nicolette Richer, DSocSci, is not just a book; it is a beacon of hope, a guide to reclaiming our health, and a testament to the extraordinary healing power that lies within the simple act of eating real, whole foods.

We live in a world where a lot of what we eat is highly processed; we stuff ourselves with food with refined oil, refined salt, refined sugar, cheese, artificial stuff—you name it. And guess what? More and more people are dealing with serious health issues, like diabetes, arthritis, and cancer. We are in a chronic disease epidemic, but Dr. Nicolette Richer emerges as a guiding light, urging us to reconsider everything we thought we knew about the connection between food and our well-being.

I've had my health wake-up call when my mom got diagnosed with colon cancer. It got me digging into the reasons behind it. And you know what I found out? Animal protein wasn't just linked to colon cancer but also a bunch of other diseases. That discovery led me to create a movement called "Badass Vegan" and launch my first book, *Badass Vegan: Fuel Your Body, Ph*ck the System*, and Live Your Life. I became a plant-based eater when I saw how the conventional American diet was utterly failing our communities. Heart disease, type 2 diabetes, high blood pressure, and chronic pain are killing Black people faster than any gun.

This big revelation also urged me to team up with the maker of the award-winning What The Health documentary team to create our joint venture, *They're Trying to Kill Us*, where I explored why people of color in America face higher rates of chronic diseases. It's a tough story about food, disease, injustice, poverty, racism, messed-up systems, and how some big companies are making loads of money while people get sick.

So, when I heard about Dr. Nicolette Richer and her mission to educate and transform lives, it hit home. She's been at it for more than two decades, helping people worldwide take control of their health and kick chronic diseases to the curb. That's what makes her work and this book so important. Her mission, much like mine, goes beyond transforming individuals physically, mentally, and spiritually. It extends to challenging the social injustices embedded in our food systems, recognizing the disproportionate impact of chronic diseases on BIPOC communities, and addressing the systemic issues that contribute to this health crisis.

Now, let's get into *Eat Real to Heal*. This book is a game-changer because it shows us how food can be our medicine. Dr. Nicolette Richer isn't just any nutrition expert or a health guru; she's the real deal. She has been a chronic disease-reversal specialist for over two decades. She started the Green Moustache, which is a collection of 100% organic, unprocessed, whole-food, delicious cafes. She's the brains behind the Richer Health Retreat Center and she's been coaching and empowering clients through her company, Richer Health Consulting, Ltd. And on top of all that, Nicolette founded a nonprofit organization, Sea to Sky Thrivers Society, to work with BIPOC communities, physicians, and youth to relearn the power of plant-based, whole-food medicine to reverse chronic lifestyle diseases.

Her experience and passion shine through every page. Nicolette keeps it really simple. She believes in the power of nature's goodies—real, whole foods that can do wonders for our health. And she's not just throwing big words at you. Nope, she breaks it down in a way that everyone can understand. Science, practical advice, research, case studies, and healing stories—it's all in there. And that's why *Eat Real to Heal* is a must-read for anyone who wants to take control of their health.

Dr. Nicolette Richer doesn't just talk the talk; she walks the walk. Through her stories and guidance, she wants us all to believe that we don't have to be stuck with diseases and that chronic diseases do not need to be a life sentence. She gives us a true roadmap to healing that anyone can follow. Her energy and understanding of how our bodies work will make you want to jump on board this health train.

So, as you flip through the pages of *Eat Real to Heal*, get ready for a journey. It's not just about reading words; it's about making a change. Dr. Nicolette Richer's wisdom and excitement will light a fire in you. You'll start thinking about what you eat and how it affects your health, when most healthcare professionals say that your diet has nothing to do with your disease. You know that is not true. This book will be a kickstarter for a healthier you.

Are you up for it? Ready to join this empowering journey? *Eat Real to Heal* is your guide, and Dr. Nicolette Richer is the friendly voice cheering you on.

Stay healthy and happy. The issue of food injustice is huge and complex, but one solution is simple: wake up, rise up, and do better in your own life. Want to give the middle finger to the processed food and pharmaceutical industries that are keeping you exhausted, sick, and disempowered? Go plant-based. Read this book. Reverse your disease. Live your best life.

John W. Hood Lewis, M.B.A.
The BadAss Vegan
Film Director/Author

INTRODUCTION

My mom and grandma raised me on real food. Thanks to our African and East Indian heritage, our home was always filled with simmering stews and soups, warm baked potatoes and okra, curried veggies and whole-grain rice, and tons of fresh, crunchy salads.

We always had vegetables and fruits growing in the backyard. We rarely ate meat. Processed junk food like macaroni, canned soda, potato chips, or sugary granola bars—this stuff just wasn't part of our routine. I don't think I ate a single bite of junk food until I was in my early teens. That's when everything changed. The first and last time time my lips tasted Kraft Dinner was when I was twenty-nine-years-old—a ridiculous pregnancy craving that came back up just as fast as it went down. Clearly, my soon-to-be-born babe inside wasn't impressed.

In high school, like many teenagers, I started working and earning a bit of my own money. I wish I could say that I spent my money on educational books, or that I donated my money to noble charities. Not exactly. I spent my money on Diet Coke, Mars bars, Big Macs, and dishes of gravy-smothered poutine. Immediately, my body reacted to these toxins. I developed intensely painful PMS symptoms and terrible, embarrassing acne. Of course, I couldn't help but wonder, "Is it because of what I've been eating?"

I stopped eating junk food and, just like magic, my bloating, cramps, and zits disappeared. That's when I realized what my mom and grandma already knew—the food you put into your body has a direct impact on how you look and feel. This is common sense, of course. But sometimes, we have to experience it in order to believe it.

I graduated from high school, went to university, and pursued a career in environmental studies. Later, I went on to complete my master's in Environmental Education and Communication at Royal Roads University. I specialized in researching toxicity in the air, water, and soil, and studying the link between pollution and chronic diseases, including cancer.

Over the years, I did thousands of hours of research, wrote hundreds of papers, and reported my findings while working for non-profits and government organizations. It was exciting work, although frustrating at times. Frustrating because, even with all the knowledge we've gained about how environmental pollution can shorten our lives, many governments and companies are still doing very little to make things better. I loved my work, but most of the time, I felt powerless. I was exhausted, as I felt like I was endlessly pushing a boulder uphill—a boulder that government and corporations kept wanting to bury. Often, I'd think, "I'm just one person. Sure, I can keep reporting my findings and keep creating education programs and policies. But there's not much I can do to influence government policies and change all of these big systems if the other people within these organizations don't want to also make the changes." The bureaucracy within the places I worked was thick like smog, slow-moving like a big, leaking oil tanker, and as resistant as a thousand tons of toxic lead. I needed to do more, but I didn't know what.

When a friend was diagnosed with recurrent breast cancer, I recalled that another friend, Bill, ten years earlier, had also been diagnosed with cancer. It had been stage IV. Terminal. Things were really bad. I remember not knowing how to respond when I heard about his diagnosis and prognosis. I remember being heartbroken and frightened for him—but, rather than opting for chemotherapy, my friend did something radical: He completely transformed his eating habits. He switched to a 100 percent plant-based meal plan packed with organic veggies, fruits, and nutrient-dense juices. He did the Gerson Therapy. He fueled his body with the best possible food—straight from gardens, trees, bushes, and vines. Within a few months, his cancer markers were...*gone.* Completely gone. As if they'd never existed. Within a year, he was cancer-free. His doctors were astounded. This seventy-two-year-old man had completely healed himself using food as medicine, and he was rewarded by living twenty more years. I tried to explain the Gerson Therapy to my other recently-diagnosed friend, but failed miserably, as I really didn't know what it entailed. This is where my research transitioned and merged from environmental health to human health.

I was astounded by Bill's recovery, too, and the fact that food had the power to heal his cancerous body, let alone reverse the emperor of all maladies. It was a pivotal moment in my life and career. Years after witnessing my friend's stunning recovery, and after much research which overcame my skepticism, I quit my job in the environmental sector. I decided to dedicate the next chapter of my life to studying the nature of, and the connection between, food and disease. I want to help other people beat disease—and beat the odds—just like Bill did.

And that's what I've done.

Today, I work as an orthomolecular nutritionist, which means I study how food can be used as medicine to reduce inflammation, alleviate pain, prevent and reverse all types of life-induced chronic degenerative disease, and help people heal faster, live longer, and most importantly, live well. I'm also the founder of the Green Moustache, a collection of 100 percent organic, plant-strong, whole-food cafes, now with eight locations across Canada (and growing).

I'm on a mission to change the way people eat. It's not just a career for me. Truly, it's an obsession. Why? Because I've seen—hundreds of times—just how powerful the results can be when my clients turn to food as medicine instead of drugs.

I have clients who have come to me with blown discs and excruciating back pain, who, after switching their diets from processed junk to real food, find that their pain goes away, their discs regenerate, and they reclaim their families, their careers, and their lives.

I have clients who come to me with cancerous tumors, and after eight weeks of organic, nutrient-dense food and juicing, the tumors have shrunk by 50 percent, or in some instances, they've vanished completely.

I have clients who come to me years after they've been diagnosed with type 2 diabetes. After working with me to overhaul their kitchen and their diet, their markers normalize, and their doctors have to take them off of their medications—sometimes in as little as seven days.

I have clients who sit in my office, sobbing, totally discouraged, because all they want is to get pregnant and they're battling infertility and endometriosis. Less than one year later, they're nursing a healthy baby.

I have young clients who are scheduled to receive highly invasive surgery—like a hysterectomy—but, after radically changing their diet, their fibroids are gone in less than three months, and the surgery gets cancelled.

I have clients who are living with intense physical and emotional pain—daily migraines, arthritis, depression, anxiety, panic attacks, suicidal thoughts—and, after switching to real food, they feel a hundred times better, and they are able to ditch the meds and rebuild their lives, careers, and relationships.

Almost every time, their doctors are stunned. "This is incredible. Such a big change. How did this happen?" they ask.

Well, it's pretty simple.

It happened because food—real, whole, diverse, nutrient-rich, garden-grown food, not processed and refined junk food—is a powerful form of medicine. And for many people living with a chronic degenerative disease, it may be the only form of medicine that will help them, not just manage their disease, but reverse it entirely.

Food can be toxic, or food can be healing, depending on what you decide to eat. This is common sense, right? When you put processed food into your body, you feel lethargic and bloated, and you interfere with your body's natural ability to heal. When you switch to clean, unprocessed, nutritious, high-quality food, you feel better and heal faster. It's just that simple. If this isn't common sense right now, then this book will teach you how to make it so.

When it comes to healing with food—if you weren't raised in a society or held in a community where food is considered medicine—then you'll simply have to make the switch to clean real food and experience its healing benefits yourself.

We can't always control how governments, big businesses, and the food industry operate, or how they're harming the environment, or how quickly or slowly they decide to make positive changes. But there is one thing we do have control over—we can control what we eat.

Only you can control what goes into your mouth; therefore, you have a great deal of control over your health. It's time to take all of this power back into your own hands.

How Do You Want to Feel?

Really think about this question.

Do you want to feel awake, alive, and strong? Do you want to feel active and fit? Do you want to feel clear-minded and focused? Do you want to feel so energized that you can do and accomplish anything you want? Do you want to feel like you're taking excellent care of your body—the one and only body you've got?

Do you want to live long enough to see your kids and grandkids get married? Do you want to feel deep joy and make memories—cycling, skiing, hiking, laughing with friends, traveling and having adventures? Do you want to feel vibrant, with plenty of energy for everything you want to do?

If you want to feel like that, it all starts with the food you put into your body.

It's time, right now, to decide how you want to feel.

And then, let's make a series of changes so you can feel that way.

This book is exactly the right place to start.

Is This for You?

Eat Real to Heal is the right book for you if...

+ You've been diagnosed with an illness, like an autoimmune disorder, infertility, heart disease, diabetes, depression, obesity, anxiety, or cancer— and you want to power up your immune system, restore your metabolism, regenerate your tissues and organs, and give your body every possible advantage in the healing process.

+ You have other non-life-threatening (but annoying) diseases like rosacea, eczema, psoriasis, or acne, and you want to see improvements.

+ You are living with chronic pain, like arthritis, back pain, headaches, migraines, gut discomfort, restless legs, and you want to have this pain disappear for good.

+ You've been relying on medication to manage your symptoms, and you'd love to kick the meds and never have to take them again. (No more pills, and no more unwanted side effects!)

+ You've had cancer in the past and you're in remission, but your body has been weakened by chemo, radiation, or surgery. You want to fuel yourself with the best possible food so you can heal faster.

+ You've witnessed your loved ones suffering— arthritis, dementia, Alzheimer's, obesity, all kinds of health issues—and you want to take preventive action. You want to protect yourself from developing those same diseases now, or further down the road.

+ You haven't been diagnosed with any specific illness, but you just don't feel great. You feel tired, lethargic, bloated, just not your best. You'd like to feel much better.

+ You already lead a fairly healthy lifestyle, but you're ready for an upgrade. You want to feel even better. You're aiming for optimum health, not just pretty good health.

+ You see people on social media and TV sipping colorful veggie juices, hiking in nature, and doing yoga poses, smiling, glowing with radiant health, and you think, "I want that life!"

If you fall into any of those categories, then this book is for you.

PS: If you are feeling blue or depressed, suffer from pre- or post-partum depression, are taking sleeping pills, or are thinking about taking your own life, then this book is definitely for you. Before reading further, contact our office, and one of our team members will give you the time and information you need so you can start experiencing mental clarity within as little as a few days.

What You'll Learn

In this book, I'll teach you how to:

+ Revamp your eating habits and your lifestyle.

+ Flood your body with nutrients and detoxify your system.

+ Boost your immune system and turn your body into a disease-fighting machine.

+ Build a health-promoting and disease-reversing kitchen and get rid of your disease-promoting kitchen.

Our goal is to get you feeling vibrant, strong, and energized, and give you the best possible chance at preventing and beating all kinds of chronic diseases—from acne to diabetes to cancer.

As you may have noticed, this book isn't about helping you manage your disease and live with your symptoms. It's about teaching you what you need to do to eliminate them for good.

What You'll Need

To follow the principles in this book, you will need:

+ A water filtration system, like a water distiller or Berkey filter, because we don't want you drinking contaminated water.

+ A juicer that's sturdy and easy to clean. I love my Norwalk juicer, but if that's too pricey for your budget, there are lots of other options. I have several recommendations on page 108 of this book.

+ A strong, easy-to-clean blender like the Vitamix or Blendtec.

+ Stainless-steel pots and pans with water/airtight lids

+ Food mill (for soup)

+ Citrus reamer

+ Sharp kitchen knives

+ Several pounds of organic, free-trade, coarsely-ground coffee, light to medium roast.

+ A coffee enema kit, including a stainless-steel (the better option) or the traditional plastic bucket, silicone tubing, a silicone enema bulb, and a set of washable tips. Google "Gerson Therapy coffee enema kit" to find one. You can get the entire kit on Amazon.com or Gerson.org for less than thirty dollars, or from Richer Health.

+ A couple of old towels and blankets and a comfy pillow.

+ A yoga mat, or some other space in your home where you can do some gentle stretching, exercise, meditation, and breathwork.

+ Fresh lemon juice, organic white vinegar, and microfiber cotton cloths, which are non-toxic options for cleaning your home.

+ And, most importantly, a kitchen that's stocked with organic fruits, vegetables, healthy grains, and oils. You'll definitely want: potatoes, tomatoes, onions, collard greens, leafy greens, squashes, apples, carrots, bananas, lemons, organic oats, maple syrup (or honey or molasses), apple cider vinegar, flax oil, and fresh herbs like parsley, cilantro, and basil, for starters. I encourage my clients to eat thirty different types of fruits and veggies every week. We want abundance and diversity! See the lists of foods to eat in abundance, foods to eat in moderation, and foods to avoid on page 188.

✦ There are a couple of other gadgets that you can invest in later, if you like, but don't worry about those right now. Stick to the items listed above, and you're ready to go!

Five Things to Know

Before you dive into this book, here are five things to know...

1. **Eating real food will change your life.**

   Every single aspect of your life is about to get a major upgrade. Exciting, right?

   When you eat real food, you sleep more deeply. You experience less inflammation and pain. Your skin becomes clearer. If you're battling a disease, your body will be fully equipped to fight back and heal. The more real food you eat, the better you feel.

2. **Real food is not fussy and complicated.**

   It's the opposite of complicated. It's simple. Whenever I use the term "real food," I'm talking about food that is clean, organic, nutrient-dense, and unprocessed. Food that grows directly from the soil, bushes, vines, and trees. Simple food. Pure food. The food your body was designed to enjoy.

3. **Switching to real food doesn't mean you're sacrificing flavor.**

    This is a common misconception. Real food doesn't have to be boring and bland. It can be absolutely delicious! Our beautiful planet has been carefully crafted to offer us an incredible diversity of colorful and tasty foods to fuel and heal our bodies. It is estimated that humans can eat nearly three hundred thousand plant species on Earth, yet, in Western industrialized nations like North America, we consume fewer than two hundred species. Even worse, we get half of our plant-sourced protein from rice and wheat. Read Warren's *The Nature of Crops* to learn more about how we've come to eat the plants we do.

    Since the industrial revolution, we've been coerced by the fake-food industry to the point where we are physically and mentally addicted to processed foods that cause disease. Similar to cigarettes, illegal drugs and alcohol, we are addicted to the chemicals in processed refined foods. However, there's a way to break the addiction, and that's by doing everything outlined in this book. This will reboot your brain, rebuild the 140 quadrillion members of your microbiome, and recharge and regenerate your mitochondria and metabolism. Even more amazing, by following the principles in this book, your taste buds will regrow, and, even if you didn't grow up eating or even liking the textures and tastes of real whole foods, your palate will start to appreciate and love them—and will even crave them.

    For breakfast, perhaps you'd like to have a big, beautiful bowl of slow-cooked oats with stewed fruits. You can even add some bright, freshly pressed orange or grapefruit juice.

For lunch and dinner, maybe a delightful and large mixed green salad with shredded carrots, beets and cabbage, drizzled with a cilantro-lime vinaigrette? Or a baked potato topped with crunchy veggies and a zesty, garlicky homemade herb dressing? Add a big, comforting bowl of stewed veggies, a savory kidney cleanse soup, and a trio of herbed baked veggies. Sounds delicious, right?

For dessert, you can enjoy a soft, crumbly dish of baked apples with cinnamon, nutmeg, a dash of maple syrup, and a scoop of banana ice cream. Yum.

Throughout this book, you'll see that real food can be tantalizing and satisfying. You're not sacrificing flavor. You're simply upgrading your ingredients for the best of the best.

4. **This is not a "diet." It's a lifelong promise.**

A "diet" (like a "weight loss diet") is a temporary plan. You follow the plan for a while, but, ultimately, you feel deprived and frustrated, and you decide, "OK, this diet is over!" You fall back into old eating habits. You've probably gotten into this pattern several times, right? Did you know that studies show that 97 percent of dieters regain everything they lost and more within three years? Diets are wonderful for emergency health situations, but are rarely the answer for general health and wellness.

It's time to break that pattern. It's time for a permanent shift, not a temporary one.

I want you to switch to real food for the rest of your life, not just for a couple of weeks. What I'm recommending in this book is not a "quick-fix diet." It's a lifelong promise. You're saying, "I promise to fuel my body with the best possible fuel, every day, for the rest of my life." Why? Because you are worth it.

Does this mean you can never eat a Kit Kat or Aero candy bar ever again? Does this mean Cheetos are off-limits forever and ever? Look, if you want to enjoy a Wunderbar once in a blue moon, I don't recommend it, but I can't stop you. If you absolutely must have it, then have it, and enjoy it. Just know that processed food has consequences—sometimes small consequences, and sometimes big ones. Similar to how most drug and alcohol addicts couldn't kick their addiction on a moderation plan or by adopting "cheat" Sundays, I recommend you take the cold-turkey approach. Evidence shows that processed foods are just as addictive as cigarettes, alcohol and the strongest prescribed and non-prescription drugs. It's time to break the cycle, kick the habit, and step into your new life of health and well-being.

Here's some great news, though: Once you switch to real food, you'll notice that your preferences change. After about two weeks, your taste buds regenerate. The junk food that used to taste amazing suddenly tastes like... blech. Garbage. A salt lick that even a cow wouldn't touch. Death even. You won't have the same cravings that you have right now.

Bottom line: We all have to ask ourselves, "What's more important to me: the fifteen-second pleasure of eating a Cadbury candy bar, or my health?" I hope you'll decide that your health—your life, your one and only life—is more precious than a rectangle of refined sugar.

5. **Food is important, but it's not everything.**

When you upgrade your eating habits, the shift is immediate and profound. Within one week, you'll feel changes—you'll start to feel better. Within two to three weeks, you'll start looking different. Within a month, your blood tests and lab results can reflect all kinds of positive changes. So much can change in a short span of time. You will be amazed.

Of course, food isn't everything. However, according to the research, food is roughly 90 percent of the cause of your health problems. The goal is to upgrade every aspect of your lifestyle, not just food. This means finding ways to de-stress and clear your mind. Moving your body every day. Walking. Breathing deeply. Drinking plenty of water. Getting a full night's rest (which will come naturally when you follow the principles in this book). Connecting with loved ones face-to-face, not just on a digital screen. Becoming a savvy patient and taking an active role in your story, not just being a passive bystander.

With every upgrade you make, you'll look and feel better. Your body will say, "thank you" in a thousand different ways.

LEGAL DISCLAIMER

This book will teach you how to use food—fruits, vegetables, some grains, and a few key supplements—as medicine so that you can prevent and reduce your risk factors for disease and lead a healthier, happier life.

However, this book is for informational purposes only, and does not constitute medical advice. Please do not use this book as a substitute for professional medical advice, diagnosis, or treatment.

Always seek the advice of a physician—or another qualified health provider—with any questions you may have regarding a medical condition. In the event of a medical emergency, call a doctor or 911 immediately. Always use common sense and listen to your body. If you sense that something isn't right, take action.

However, if you are like a recent client of mine, who is less than thirty years old and was diagnosed with cancer and scheduled for the removal of major organ systems, suffers from a history of chronic health conditions, and was told by an oncologist not to give up smoking and definitely not to change to a plant-strong diet and lifestyle—well, just go ahead and tell your doctor, "You are FIRED!" and get yourself a second and third opinion. You are allowed to do that. And find a doctor who has more than the allocated two hours of nutritional training given in most medical schools.

PART ONE:

The New Era of Health— Empowerment Through Eating Real

You Are Not Alone—I've Got You

I know that dealing with chronic illness can feel incredibly lonely—like you are lost in a labyrinth with no way out. But you're not alone and you are not lost. You are exactly where you are supposed to be, here, right now, reading this book and learning that there is another way. That *yes!* It is possible to live free of your chronic conditions.

And I get it—the constant struggles, the endless doctors' appointments, the financial strain, and the worries about the future. Then there's the frustration and complexities of managing multiple treatments, not to mention the scary side-effects of multiple medications. It's tough.

Then there's the confusion arising from conflicting nutritional advice out there, which can be downright overwhelming. Through my own personal health challenges and from direct experience with thousands of clients from around the world, these are all burdens I recognize all too closely.

I understand how you might be feeling adrift, lost in a sea of uncertainty. I've been there too, in emergency rooms with my daughters, feeling isolated and desperate for genuine support. But here, within these pages, you've found a safe space. I've been through similar battles, and I'm here to walk this journey with you.

I know that the persistent symptoms you are facing cast shadows over your days and limit your ability to thrive daily. So, let's face this challenge together, like two comrades on a shared mission—your vibrant, chronic-disease-free life. Know that you are one step closer to figuring it out—to finding that path to healing and hope. You're not alone—not anymore.

Welcome to *Eat Real to Heal* 2.0

I'm bursting with gratitude as I introduce the second edition of *Eat Real to Heal.* Your support and engagement since the first edition has been the driving force behind this journey. The healing stories that our readers shared with me from around the world after the first edition came out inspired me profoundly. Know this: I almost didn't publish the first edition of *Eat Real to Heal.* You see, days before our publishers were about to hit the print button, I remember standing in a Starbucks bookstore amid a sea of books, feeling nauseous to my core, questioning—"Does the world need yet another book on nutrition?" Thank goodness I didn't listen to the self-sabotaging voice, and since then my reader's voices and responses to my first book silenced my doubts and reaffirmed the book's purpose—to change and save lives.

The actions taken as a result of my book have had a tremendous impact on dozens of continents, from North America to Europe, from Africa to Australia and beyond. Hundreds—maybe even thousands—of chronic conditions like endometriosis, heart problems, diabetes, MS and other autoimmune disorders, and even cancer have been reversed thanks to my readers' determination and lifestyle changes. Your generosity in sharing your transformations not only changed your own lives, but also served as guiding lights for others. Our *Eat Real to Heal* podcast—a platform where we've shared wisdom, healing stories, research and hope—has reached ears globally, thanks to your overwhelming support.

This second edition—*Eat Real to Heal: Using Food to Live Healthier*—is more than a book; it's a continued movement toward human and planetary healing. And I am even more committed to empowering you with practical tools and insights. Your commitment to wellness aligns perfectly with the principles within these pages. By embracing these ideas and putting them into practice, you're not just transforming your own life—you're becoming a beacon of hope and light for others battling chronic diseases.

If you read our first book, I want to express my profound thanks. If you implemented the methods and healed yourself, I invite you to share your journey on our podcast. Your experiences can inspire others, instilling hope in those facing similar challenges. Your choice to heal doesn't just transform your world; it creates ripples of inspiration throughout our global community. Together, let's pave the way to a future where chronic diseases are a thing of the past.

Thank you for being part of this transformative movement. Here's to our collective journey toward optimal health, vitality, and a future filled with wellness.

You Haven't Tried *Everything*

I often hear the same objection from the people who reach out to me: "I've tried everything; nothing works." Yet, when I ask if they've ever attempted a holistic approach rooted in 100% organic, plant-based, whole foods—nothing processed or packaged, straight from farm to table— paired with essential supplements from a compounding pharmacy, the answer is almost always no. It's about embracing nutrient-rich foods, all their goodness retained, complemented by century-old vegetable juice recipes and regular liver detoxes, all from the comfort of your home.

The surprising truth? In just seven to twenty-one days, my clients often find themselves feeling markedly better. A few more weeks and blood results show that inflammatory markers return to normal. Within twelve weeks, HbA1C levels return to prediabetic and often normal range and insulin resistance is a thing of the past. Arthritis pain— gone without medications. Even if you are one of my rare

3 percent of client cases where slight adjustments are needed—I've found that all you may need is a little extra lysine and NAC+ if you have high Epstein-Barr virus levels or a MTHFR gene mutation, or perhaps extra vitamin A if you have a determined genetic beta-carotene conversion issue—the foundation remains: real food, an abundance and diversity of whole food nutrients, and robust daily liver support.

My question is: are you ready to try this, even if there's a chance it might not work? Consider the alternative: a life of non-organic, processed foods; neglecting your liver; and sipping on modern, sugary drinks that are slowly but surely harming us. It's time to go back to basics, to eat as our ancestors did, and reclaim the health they enjoyed—a life free from the epidemic rates of chronic diseases that people are living with today... Well, only the people who choose or are forced[1] to consume a Standard American Diet (SAD). More on that later in this book. So, are you willing to embrace this movement toward a vibrant, healthy life? Let's embark on this transformative journey together.

The Mighty Potato— Where Did We Go Wrong?

Let's talk about a trend that's affected a number of us—the rise of low-carb, high-protein diets, often known as keto or Atkins. In the 80s and 90s, these diets gained massive popularity, but the impact has been far from positive. Here's where the problem lies: these diets were originally studied for epilepsy patients in the short term. But somehow, this approach became a mainstream solution for everyone, perpetuated by the media, self-proclaimed nutrition experts, and health practitioners who lacked deep scientific knowledge about the intricacies of these diets and their

---

1 Regarding choice vs being *forced* to consume the Standard American Diet, please read the section on Food Nutrition Deserts.

surrounding research methods.

I've seen the fallout in my clients who followed keto for months. What happened? Insulin resistance cropped up due to excessive animal fats and proteins, neuropathy developed from clogged microcapillaries, and mental health suffered because their brains lacked the vital nutrients found in phyto-nutrient rich whole high-carb foods. The concerning part? Most practitioners advocating keto didn't present the complete story. Long-term human studies were scarce, and the few available revealed alarming outcomes: higher rates of clinical depression, heart disease, stroke, and autoimmune conditions among long-term keto followers.

Now we have a chance to set things right. Some of you might be thinking, "I lost weight on keto, so what's the issue?" The real question is about your overall health. What's happening inside your arteries? How's your insulin resistance? Are you planning on keto for life? How's your pancreas and liver holding up? These are critical questions. We're not just individual cases; our choices affect entire populations. Research spanning decades consistently shows that societies thriving on plant-based, low-animal-fat, and healthy protein-level diets live longer and healthier lives, meaning they suffer less from chronic illnesses and they live longer—who wouldn't want that?

This is the goal we should all be reaching for: a long, disease-free life. Currently, as early as three years old in many cases, humans are facing chronic diseases, from diabetes to arthritis, often leading to a lifetime of medications, treatments, surgeries, and expensive alternative and often unproven therapies.

Did you know that in the United States and Canada, one in four adults suffers from arthritis or related conditions? Arthritis is fully preventable and reversible at any age, yet millions are put on prescriptions with numerous side effects, leading to a cycle of more medications and escalating costs. The situation isn't limited to adults; even young children are now diagnosed with juvenile idiopathic arthritis, a condition called "idiopathic" because the cause remains a "mystery" among doctors not trained in nutrition.

There's hope, though. In Ep. 26 with Suzanne Meadows on our *Eat Real to Heal* podcast, you'll learn how this mother used food as medicine to permanently heal her son who was diagnosed with juvenile idiopathic arthritis. The fact that only one identical twin suffered from it raises intriguing questions about genes versus environment. Stories like Suzanne's son drive us to rethink our approach to eating and living. It's time to shift from harmful trends to holistic health, where our choices empower us and the generations to come.

 For a deeper understanding of the concepts discussed in this book and to learn more about reversing juvenile idiopathic arthritis, I encourage you to listen to Susannah Meadows' TEDx talk which can be found here: https://www.ted.com/talks/susannah_meadows_confronting_chronic_disease_and_refusing_to_give_up[2]

This is why I'm writing this book—to share a profound solution, a method that goes beyond trends and empty promises. It's about empowering you with knowledge, guiding you toward a path where chronic diseases are not just managed, but truly reversed. In the pages that follow, I'll unveil the Eat Real to Heal program, a revolutionary approach rooted in science and compassion. It's not just another diet—it's a lifestyle, a way of embracing food as a healer, as a tool for reclaiming your health and vitality. So, stay with me as we dive into the heart of the matter, exploring the true keys to reversing chronic diseases and fostering a life of enduring well-being.

2 Centers for Disease Control and Prevention, 2020
Centers for Disease Control and Prevention, 2021

Unmasking the True Wealth: Your Health

Recently, I found myself speaking at a boogie event, surrounded by millions of dollars of extravagance: designer clothes, sparkling jewelry, glamorous handbags, and the telltale signs of a *lot* of plastic surgery. What struck me was the jarring absence of knowledge in the room about the profound impact of food as medicine. In this sea of affluence, health, our most priceless possession, seemed forgotten.

The aftermath of the event was sadly predictable. A slew of emails and calls flooded in, each one laden with diagnoses and health woes. It became painfully apparent that even amidst luxury, ignorance about health prevailed. Shockingly, this scenario isn't unique. It echoes a broader truth: a staggering 60% of our population grapples with chronic degenerative diseases and these rates are as prevalent among the rich as the poor. Collectively—despite the varying numbers on our tax returns, we are oblivious to the transformative power of proper nutrition.

While wealth affords better food and education, it rarely guides individuals toward the right choices in chronic disease reversal, metabolic nutrition, and detoxification. Perhaps, the allure of expensive wines, steaks, and seafood blinds them to the profound impact of their choices. However, the old adage rings true: when it comes to health, you either invest in it now or pay for it later.

Remember, all the riches in the world hold no value on your deathbed. Your true wealth lies in the vitality of your body and the richness of your health. It's time to shift the focus, invest wisely, and embrace the ultimate luxury: vibrant, enduring health.

My Purpose and Mission

I wrote this book to spark a revolution where every reader actively participates in their healing journey. Since the first edition in 2018, *Eat Real to Heal* has grown into impactful initiatives, including the 22 Million Strong campaign. We aim to empower twenty-two million individuals by 2030, representing 10% of North Americans battling reversible chronic illnesses. I've witnessed the powerful domino effect—one person's healing inspiring at least ten others. This ripple effect, reminiscent of Malcolm Gladwell's theory, is our strategy to end the chronic disease epidemic. We're not just a campaign; we're a force, determined to transform health narratives for millions. Join us.

I wish for this book to be a beacon of hope and wisdom amid modern health challenges. Its purpose is clear: to demonstrate the transformative power of embracing a real, unprocessed, whole-food-based lifestyle. I share lessons from ancestral wisdom, travel, and personal experience to guide you toward optimal health. My aim is to help you understand the vital link between nutrition, detoxification, and chronic diseases. Through science-backed insights, practical advice, and inspiring stories, this book serves as a roadmap to better health. It's more than facts; it's a lifeline for those breaking free from chronic illnesses, empowering you to reclaim control over your health and life. My deepest hope is that you discover the profound impact food and detoxification can have, and find the pathway to vibrant living within these pages.

Returning to the Motherland

Shortly after *Eat Real to Heal* version 1.0, a profound journey unfolded, leading me back to the roots of my heritage, in the heart of Chiradzulu, Malawi, Africa. In the very village where generations of my family had lived for centuries, I reconnected with a way of life that seemed almost ancient amidst our modern, hectic world. During my visit, I had the incredible privilege of harvesting food alongside my beloved grandma, whom I hadn't seen since my childhood. Together, we gathered an array of fresh produce—dark leafy greens, beans, peas, potatoes, onions, and garlic—from gardens that surrounded our family's thatched roof huts. What struck me profoundly was not just the simplicity of our meals, but their innate wisdom.

In Chiradzulu, traditional Malawian dishes were prepared with the most basic of methods: the Long and Low approach, utilizing minimal water. Pit cooking techniques synonymous to Indigenous pit cooking methods are also used there. We pounded maize, the staple corn of Malawi, into flour to create *nsima*, a nourishing porridge. In this ancient village, devoid of the trappings of modern processed foods, something astounding stood out: there wasn't an ounce of refined salt, sugar, or oil within hundreds of miles and therefore none could be added to our meals.

These highly refined, toxic ingredients are virtually absent from their lives and animal fats and proteins are kept to a minimum, and my family members—who are at risk under the threat of infectious diseases—thrive well into their 90s, Blue Zone style. To my family in our remote Africa village, refined foods are alien. They have yet to find their way into their culinary traditions, though soy- and corn-oil-producing companies like Nestle are trying desperately to influence all of Africa to adopt our ridiculous Western ways—as seen by the mass marketing and billboards visible roadside in the more urban centers.

This realization sparked the genesis of my new venture, our Decolonizing Your Plate online course, a transformative six-week journey inspired by the pure, unadulterated wisdom of my ancestors. As we explore this further in the upcoming pages of this edition, we'll delve into the positive and negative effects of colonization; the magic behind decolonized meals, untangling the intricate web of history and nutrition; and paving the way for a return to a simpler, healthier method of nourishing our bodies and souls.

That's when it hit me that the therapy that I teach my clients, the Eat Real to Heal program—which is based on the Gerson Therapy principles of 100% organic, unrefined, plant-based, whole-food, processed-salt-sugar-and-oil-free—exemplifies the way that my maternal relatives have eaten their whole lives. It's what kept them free of chronic diseases for centuries, and it's what helps my clients reverse their chronic diseases. Let's see what we can learn from them.

Ten Lessons from COVID-19

In the midst of the global COVID-19 pandemic, we all realized how crucial our health truly is. Those with underlying health conditions and comorbidities like heart disease, diabetes, and other autoimmune disorders faced higher COVID risks and even rates of death, alerting the public to the fact that we need to build up our health resilience. We also found that catching COVID with existing high inflammatory conditions and other metabolic diseases made you more susceptible to virus-related complications.

Now more than ever, we understand that good health starts with the nutrients—the building blocks of our cells, tissues, bones, organs, and more—that we put into our bodies. Organic, unprocessed, whole foods have taken the spotlight, showing us that what we eat can be the best medicine. This shift has led us back to an era in which nutrition and detoxification are fundamental in fighting chronic diseases.

Startling statistics from Health Canada and the CDC show that only three out of ten people eat enough fruits and vegetables on a daily basis. This gap in our nutrition emphasizes the urgent need for education and action. Fortunately, small grass-roots communities are coming together to embrace the healing power of whole foods. Through education and accessible resources, people are learning how to harness nature's nourishment to reverse chronic diseases and improve their well-being. This change not only promises healthier lives but also marks a significant shift in our healthcare approach, where food and detoxification are seen as essential agents of healing and prevention.

Here are some important lessons we learned from the pandemic:

+ Immune Resilience: Building a strong immune system through a balanced diet, exercise, and stress management became crucial.

+ Chronic Inflammation: Prioritizing anti-inflammatory foods and lifestyle choices became vital for overall health, considering the risks of chronic inflammation.

+ Plant-Powered Diets: Plant-based nutrition, rich in vitamins and antioxidants, became essential in strengthening our bodies.

+ Mind-Body Connection: Mental health's impact on physical well-being became evident. Practices like meditation and yoga proved invaluable in reducing stress and supporting overall mental and physical health.

+ Natural Approaches: People sought natural ways

to boost health, leading to a reduced reliance on prescription medications. Nutrition and lifestyle changes became proactive measures.

✦ Hygiene Practices: Regular handwashing and cleanliness became ingrained habits, reducing the risk of various infections.

✦ Telemedicine: Many couldn't get in to see their primary practitioners, resulting in easier access to healthcare professionals via telemedicine, which could promote increased regularity in check-ups, preventive care, and early detection of health issues. However, more work is needed to strike a balance between in-person and telemedicine.

✦ Respiratory Health: Awareness about lung health increased, emphasizing the importance of avoiding smoking, improving indoor air quality, and regular exercise.

✦ Community Support: While the pandemic divided families and friends, the pandemic also highlighted the prevalence of mental health struggles and the need for community as many were left suffering in isolation. We value, more than ever, the importance of real, face-to-face social connections as well as the need to support each other emotionally, spiritually, and mentally more than ever before.

✦ Preventive Healthcare: Finally, I witnessed a focus shift toward preventive healthcare, making regular exercise, balanced nutrition, and stress management necessary components of a healthy lifestyle.

These lessons have reshaped our perspective, emphasizing the value of a holistic approach to health and well-being. More importantly, the pandemic showed us that we can't take our health for granted, as all it can takes is one virus to come along and take the planet out at the knees.

But wait... it's essential to grasp the broader context of health risks, especially in the face of alarming statistics like those surrounding COVID-19. While the pandemic has tragically claimed the lives of roughly 6.8 million people worldwide as of October 2023, it's crucial to recognize that cardiovascular diseases (CVDs) pose a persistent and significant threat to global health. These diseases, including heart attacks and strokes, continue to be the leading cause of death worldwide, claiming a staggering 17.9 million lives *every year!* This statistic underscores the importance of focusing on our overall heart health, making lifestyle choices that reduce the risk of cardiovascular diseases. While the fight against COVID-19 remains vital, understanding the ongoing prevalence of conditions like CVDs, diabetes, arthritis, and other common and life-threatening diseases is essential to implementing the proactive measures necessary to maintain our health and well-being in the long run.

Are We Making Progress?

Isn't it incredible how the world is shifting? Our medical community is transforming, embracing the profound potential of plant-based, whole foods. There are more plant-forward doctors, nutritionists, and healthcare warriors who are shifting from being solely pill-pushers to lifestyle medicine experts. They've become guides, leading people away from disease, medication, and surgery. I believe that we are witnessing a health revolution right now, a revolution rooted in the ancient wisdom of Ayurveda and Traditional Chinese medicine, and bolstered by the knowledge from over sixty-eight thousand studies since 2019.

But here's the reality check: despite this progress, we're still drowning in chronic diseases. If your doctor isn't open to the fact that these diseases are reversible, it's time for a serious conversation or even a change. We've got this incredible knowledge base, spanning centuries of traditional wisdom and current cutting-edge research.

Consuming nutritious, unprocessed, whole food while minimizing human made toxins in our lives is our most potent medicine, a truth echoed not only by scientific studies but also by the ancient healers who came before us.

So, let's raise our voices. Let's demand a healthcare system that recognizes the transformative power of food. Let's be the driving force behind a future where chronic diseases are not just managed but reversed. We hold this power within us; it's time to use it. Together, let's script a new narrative in healthcare, one where vibrant health is not a luxury but a fundamental right.

$3.9 Trillion Gone Each Year

It's astounding to consider that in North America, a staggering $3.9 trillion is spent each year treating fully preventable *and* reversible chronic diseases. Let me repeat that — *North American taxpayers spend 3.9 TRILLION dollars each year*, which account for 97% of our collective 4.3 *trillion*-dollar healthcare spending budget, on surgeries, medications, and other treatments for people with diabetes, MS, heart diseases, infertility, gut health issues, arthritis and other autoimmune disorders, and more. And we are spending this money in spite of the fact that we have *all* the scientific proof that we'll ever need to prove that we can eradicate these conditions quickly and easily. This allocation of resources is nothing short of absurd. Every year, countless lives are lost due to the shortcomings of a medical, pharmaceutical, educational, and food production system that, in reality, promotes a culture of sick care rather than genuine healthcare.

The tragedy lies not just in the enormous financial burden, but in the human cost we endure. What makes this situation even more frustrating is the knowledge that this dire scenario could be drastically different. Imagine a world where our medical professionals are adequately trained in the crucial role of nutrition and detoxification in health and healing.

It's astonishing that most doctors receive less than four hours of nutrition training throughout their eight years of medical training, despite their genuine interest and desire to learn the subject. The gap between what our healthcare system could be and what it currently is highlights the urgent need for a profound transformation—one that empowers doctors with the knowledge they need to prevent and reverse diseases, making healthcare truly about health and not just sickness management.

Now let's imagine…what if we redirected the staggering $3.9 trillion currently spent on treating preventable diseases? We could channel these resources into transformative avenues that significantly enhance lives. First and foremost, investing in mental health services that are effective and accessible would create a robust support system for those in need. Additionally, allocating funds toward research and development for rare genetic conditions would pave the way for breakthrough treatments and therapies, offering hope to individuals and families facing these challenges. Moreover, enhancing research and development initiatives for people with mobility challenges could lead to innovations in assistive technologies, empowering individuals to lead more independent lives. Furthermore, dedicating resources to preventive healthcare measures, public health education, and promoting healthier lifestyles could drastically reduce the prevalence of preventable diseases, saving both lives and financial resources in the long run. By focusing on these areas, we can foster a healthier, more inclusive society and improve the overall well-being of countless individuals.

Doctor and Nurse Suicide Rates

In my experiences training physicians across continents, in places as diverse as China, the USA, and Canada, I've witnessed something deeply troubling. These dedicated healers, whom we entrust with our well-being, have borne their souls to me. In hushed tones, they've shared heart-wrenching stories of their own battles with overwhelming stress, depression, and even attempts at suicide, stemming from their profound frustration and trauma within our healthcare system. They've rolled up their sleeves, revealing wrists that bear the scars of their struggles. What's even more heartbreaking is that many of these physicians, despite their medical expertise, find themselves battling debilitating chronic diseases with no clear path to reversal. Why? Because they, too, are caught in the web of nutritional misinformation that plagues our society. Check out these stats:

+ Physicians have a suicide rate twice as high as the general population.

+ Nurses, both male and female, face an increased risk of suicide based on data from the 2005–2016 National Violent Death Reporting System.

+ Globally, a beloved human commits suicide every forty seconds, as per the World Health Organization.

+ In the United States, suicide is the tenth leading cause of death, with thirteen suicides per 100,000 individuals.

+ And despite decreasing overall mortality rates, suicide rates are increasing in the US.

It's crucial to understand that this isn't merely a problem of individual doctors and nurses. No, this is a systemic issue, an affliction that taints every corner of our healthcare structure. Physicians, nurses, and patients alike are trapped within a labyrinth of confusion and despair, victims of a broken system that fails to recognize the fundamental importance of nutrition, detoxification, and preventative care. It's not about blaming doctors—it's about acknowledging the crisis within our healthcare system that demands urgent, comprehensive change. The time has come for us all to rise above this challenge, demanding a transformation that values the health of both doctors and patients, fostering a culture of true healing, understanding, and hope.

Certainly, addressing nutrition in the context of mental health is crucial for holistic well-being. It's increasingly recognized that what we eat directly impacts not only our physical health but also our mental health. Here's a breakdown of why this is important:

+ Nutrition and Mental Health: Proper nutrition impacts your mental health. Essential nutrients, like omega-3 fatty acids, vitamins, minerals, enzymes, hormones, and more, play key roles in brain function and can influence mood and behavior. Deficiencies in these nutrients are directly linked to mental health disorders like depression, anxiety, panic attacks, bipolar, and schizophrenia.

+ Toxic Chemicals in Foods: Our modern food systems often involve the use of pesticides, additives, antibiotics, dyes, fillers, and preservatives, which load your body with harmful chemicals. Thousands of studies show that ongoing daily exposure to these toxins contribute to mental health issues. Eliminating or reducing the intake of processed foods and choosing organic, pesticide-free options is a crucial and positive first step to healing yourself from mental health conditions.

+ **Gut-Brain Axis:** Emerging research emphasizes the importance of the gut-brain axis, a multi-dimensional communication system between the central nervous system and the gastrointestinal tract. A healthy gut contributes to a balanced mental state. Consuming probiotics and, more importantly, prebiotics in the form of fiber-rich foods nurtures a diverse and beneficial gut microbiota, which is directly linked to improved mood and stress management.

+ **The Need for Dialogue:** It's essential to promote awareness about the connection between nutrition and mental health. Healthcare providers, educators, and the general public need to engage in more widespread levels, in conversations about the impact of diet on mental well-being. Encouraging open discussions can help reduce the stigma associated with mental health issues and foster a culture of understanding and support.

+ **Educational Initiatives:** Education about nutrition should be an integral part of mental health initiatives in all areas of education from primary school to universities and also within workplaces. Teaching people, including patients, caregivers, and healthcare professionals, about the importance of an organic, nutrient-dense, plant-forward, whole-foods lifestyle, free from harmful chemicals, will empower individuals to make healthier food choices.

+ **Policy Changes:** Advocacy for policies that support access to affordable, nutritious, soil-to-table foods and beverages is crucial. Governments and organizations need to start working together to create environments where fresh, whole foods are accessible and affordable for everyone. This includes supporting local farmers and sustainable agriculture practices instead of spending millions subsidizing refined and processed food suppliers and the meat and dairy producers.

It's time to start integrating discussions about nutrition, eliminating toxic elements from our food systems, and nurturing our gut-brain axis at the highest level of government and within all educational institutions and businesses, really. This is a pivotal step toward fostering better mental health in our homes and communities. By acknowledging the interconnectedness of physical and mental health, we can pave the way for comprehensive healing and overall well-being, and eradicate the mental health crisis that we are all entangled in.

Food Nutrition Deserts

The crisis runs deeper than our flawed healthcare system; it's woven into the very fabric of our food production and distribution networks. Millions of individuals, particularly those from low-income backgrounds and marginalized communities, find themselves residing in what we term 'food deserts.' These are areas where access to fresh, nutritious, and affordable food is severely limited or, in some cases, entirely absent. Food deserts essentially create nutritional wastelands within our own communities, where residents struggle to find nourishing sustenance. Building upon this notion, John Lewis, the inspiring advocate from the Bad Ass Vegan community, introduced the concept of 'nutrition deserts.' In these areas, people not only lack access to healthy food but are also inundated with high-calorie, low-nutrient options, leading to what can only be described as high-calorie malnutrition. It's a haunting paradox where individuals consume an excess of calories but remain starved of essential nutrients, a crisis perpetuated by a broken system that demands immediate attention and radical reform.

But There's Hope:
Healing Hero Case Studies

Now let's dive into some actual case studies. They're filled with incredible stories of people triumphing over chronic illnesses, proving the incredible power of embracing a whole foods lifestyle. These narratives are more than just inspiring tales; they're proof that change, even in the face of tough health challenges, is not just a possibility but something achievable—even for you. As we go through these stories together, let them be a source of inspiration. Each story showcases the strength of the human spirit and the impact of informed choices. It's not just reading; it's witnessing real-life journeys that prove wellness isn't just a dream but a tangible reality waiting for us to bring it to life. Get ready to be moved, inspired, and empowered by the amazing journeys you'll find in these pages.

Type 1 Diabetes

Meet Annie—a young woman, just twenty-one, thrust into the clutches of type one diabetes after battling COVID and a subsequent outbreak of hives. She lived in fear of daunting insulin spikes and crashes. Yet, embracing our program, she defied the odds, reducing her insulin intake from eighty units to merely three, her A1c levels dropping from 7.7 to a remarkable 6. Her tale echoes a fundamental truth—the human body, armed with even one functional beta cell as determined by a C-peptide test, possesses the capacity to regenerate, defeating the ominous specters of high and low blood sugar levels. Annie is thriving, no longer facing the daily stress of her disease. And the best part of this story: she eats high-carb whole foods daily at every meal like potatoes, oatmeal, and an abundance of fruit and juices— foods that her previous health practitioners had told her to stay away from.

Anxiety, Depression, Brain Fog, and More...

Now meet Margaret, aged fifty-two. She was tormented by anxiety, brain fog, candida overgrowth, insulin resistance, debilitating gut health issues, depression, and around twenty additional symptoms. She spent thousands on functional medicine doctors, chiropractors, physiotherapists, and lab work, repeatedly being poked and prodded. Eventually, everyone said that it must be in her head, as none of the treatments were working...until she tried our Eat Real to Heal program, that is. Within five days of starting our program, she was shocked and equally relieved. The symptoms were starting to go away. One by one, they disappeared, and Margaret, for the first time in decades, had a newfound lease on life. Her brain fog lifted, the pain eased, her gut settled, her depression lessened, and her energy quadrupled. When health practitioners don't lead with total body nutrition first and daily detoxification, it's like trying to repair a leaky roof without addressing the damaged foundation at the same time—the rainwater will still get in. Without prioritizing total body nutrition and daily detoxification, health practitioners are merely addressing symptoms rather than tackling the root cause of health issues, much like fixing visible damage while ignoring the underlying structural problems. Emphasizing holistic well-being through nutrition and detoxification is fundamental for building a strong, resilient foundation for overall health and vitality.

Heart Disease & Diabetes Type 2

Then there's John and Brenda, a couple married for over 50 years, two eighty-six-year-olds confined to their chairs, once ensnared in medications. In a mere three months, they shed 90% of their medications, regaining vitality and reclaiming their farm. Another client, suffering from severe allergies and psoriasis, rediscovered a life devoid of swelling and itchiness, her psoriasis vanishing, her mental and physical health thriving.

Scleroderma & Unexplained Weight-Loss

Meet Natasha, a thirty-six-year-old client who arrived at our wellness center weighing a mere 79 lbs at 5 feet and 6 inches tall. Her skeletal appearance, gray complexion, and deteriorating mental health, characterized by intense brain fog and an inability to process information, reflected the severe toll of scleroderma and mental health challenges following two devastating car accidents. Through our tailored approach of a low-calorie, low-fat, high-fiber, nutrient-dense diet combined with daily detoxification, Natasha experienced an astounding transformation. When she left our center, she weighed 105 lbs, her complexion had regained a healthy hue from head to toe, and her mental health had markably improved. Her psychiatrist noted that her mental state was the best he had ever witnessed, marking a significant positive change from the difficult period following her accidents and subsequent autoimmune disorder diagnosis. Natasha's journey underscores the power of our approach, sparking crucial questions about nutrition and its impact on complex health conditions like scleroderma and mental disorders. We invite others to share their experiences and contribute to our ongoing quest to understand and improve lives.

Cystic Fibrosis, PCOS, Panic Attacks, and More....

Zoey, diagnosed with cystic fibrosis, defied medical expectations, enhancing her health to a point where doctors now predict a life expectancy into her eighties or ninties. Dahlia, gripped by PCOS and depression, found healing and went on to become a beacon of support herself. Cailin, plagued by PCOS, chronic pain, depression, and low energy, transformed herself into the epitome of health and went on to run her first half-marathon within three months of starting our program.

Consider also the story of twenty-two-year-old Steven, trapped in a year-long panic attack disorder. Through our program, he not only found his way to recovery but became a healer, establishing a sanctuary rooted in tradition and ecological wisdom, to offer solace to other young millennials suffering from chronic diseases and mental health disorders. His work with Indigenous communities exemplifies our collective vision: harmony with the earth, unity in healing.

And we have hundreds more healing hero clients — too many to name here. There's Michael, who reversed his rheumatoid arthritis and dropped his inflammatory markers to zero, and was able to return to playing sports and working. Amanda, who healed herself from Grave's disease, also returned to work after experiencing chronic pain for decades. Matthew, an eighty-year-old who had to stop playing music because his arthritis was crippling, after a few short months on our program, bought himself a new guitar and is back playing music with his band — devoting the rest of his life to playing shows in retirement and extended living homes for people with Alzheimer's and dementia.

You, too, can be a part of these narratives. By embracing the principles outlined in this book, you can script your own story of triumph over chronic illness. We invite you to be our next client story, a testament to the power of perseverance and transformation. Our mission, our ambitious goal of empowering twenty-two million people to reverse chronic diseases by 2030, can't be achieved alone. We call upon fellow health practitioners — doctors, chiropractors, yoga instructors, traditional Chinese medicine practitioners, naturopaths, osteopaths — to join hands with us. Let's turn this tide and usher in an era of health and vitality for millions.

Does Nutrition & Detoxification Work for *All* Chronic Conditions?

I am dedicated to helping clients improve their health through metabolic nutrition and detoxification strategies. The only conditions I do not work with are leukemias, ALS, and specific brain cancers due to intricate biological and biochemical reasons, including the necessity to manage healing reactions, necessary immune system suppression which is the opposite outcome that we are aiming for, and limited opportunities for success.

Although I haven't had the chance to work directly with clients suffering from ALS or Parkinson's, I am eager to explore the possibilities. Current research indicates that nutrition can potentially slow down the progression of these diseases, but studies haven't delved into the comprehensive hyper nutrition and detoxification methods we employ. I am open to collaborating, researching, and experimenting to determine the effectiveness of our approach. For more information, please contact us at nicolette@richerhealth.ca or schedule an introductory call. Together, let's assess if our program aligns with your specific condition and goals.

ALS Questions

Though I have had the privilege of working with clients suffering from unexplained weight loss due to scleroderma, I'm not certain how our program would fare with someone diagnosed with ALS. Despite consuming high-calorie diets rich in fats, dairy, meats, and carbohydrates, their weight loss persisted. However, a transformative shift occurred when they transitioned to a low-calorie, low-fat, high-fiber, nutrient-dense diet coupled with daily detoxification. Almost immediately, they began gaining weight, and remarkably, their chronic scleroderma symptoms regressed, eventually disappearing entirely.

This outcome has raised significant questions, particularly regarding ALS patients. Many ALS organizations advocate for high-calorie, low-nutrient diets, yet the scientific evidence supporting their effectiveness remains inconclusive. Recognizing the need for further research, we invite individuals whose family members with ALS have followed a low-calorie, high-nutrient diet to reach out. Your experiences can offer invaluable insights, contributing to our collective understanding of these complex conditions and potentially paving the way for more effective treatments. Let's join forces to unravel these mysteries and improve the lives of those affected.

The Eat Real to Heal Program: A Potato-Lined Path

"The world will heal when people are able to eat potatoes again."

—Dr. Nicolette Richer

This is a book that saves lives. And people's lives will be saved and the planet will be healed when we can all go back to eating potatoes again. Let me take you behind the scenes, to when our publishers reached out with a troubling message—books claiming to offer healing outside the realm of established medical organizations like the World Health Organization were facing censorship on platforms like Amazon. In many parts of the world, governments and organizations are cracking down on medical misinformation with policies such as California's AB 2098, YouTube's new policies announced in August of 2023 to target medical misinformation, and British Columbia's Bill 36 which is a comprehensive law that imposes strict penalties, such as two-year imprisonment, on physicians found guilty of disseminating specific forms of inaccurate or deceptive information.

This revelation hit home when our podcasts, brimming with genuine stories of individuals reversing chronic diseases, were deemed in violation of providing medical misinformation, but without any explanation of what that information was. And our podcasts don't just feature client stories; they feature scientists, medical doctors, researchers, and real people sharing their raw, unfiltered, first-hand experiences healing themselves or helping their clients and patients heal—all with diagnostic data like scans and lab work showing that they are healed. Despite this, our stories of healing are being silenced, and it was hard to wrap our heads around this reality. This saddens me because it means I won't be able to share this vital information that could save your life or the life of one of your loved ones.

Now, let's return to the essence of the Eat Real to Heal program, encapsulated by the quote, *"The world will heal when people are able to eat potatoes again."* This profound statement carries the weight of transformative potential. It signifies more than just a dietary choice; it represents a return to the fundamental, healing power of whole foods. Embracing potatoes without having your blood sugars spike embodies the very essence of genuine health. Let's break down the science in simple terms. When I say true health is being able to eat potatoes without blood sugar spikes, I'm referring to a crucial aspect of our body's functioning: insulin sensitivity.

When someone is insulin resistant, their body's cells don't respond well to insulin, a hormone that helps regulate blood sugar levels. This means when they eat foods like potatoes, which contain carbohydrates, their blood sugar levels can spike and then crash. These fluctuations can lead to various health issues, including diabetes.

However, regaining insulin sensitivity means their cells respond appropriately to insulin. When they eat potatoes, their body can efficiently process the carbohydrates without causing drastic blood sugar swings. In other words, their body is functioning optimally, keeping blood sugar levels stable and reducing the risk of health problems related to insulin resistance, such as diabetes. Achieving this balance is a significant milestone on the path to genuine health and well-being.

This method, championed in the pages of this book, isn't just a dietary approach; it's a revolutionary path to healing, a beacon of hope guiding us toward true wellness. The stories within these pages are testament to the potency of this method, reaffirming the healing prowess residing within each of us and underlining the vital importance of reclaiming our health, one potato at a time.

So why did I give this section the subtitle, "A Potato-Lined Path"? Because potatoes stand out as one of the healthiest foods on the planet, containing the right balance of proteins, fats, fiber, micro-nutrients, macro-nutrients, and starches (both resistant and non-resistant). Despite their nutritional richness, medical misinformation in the world of nutrition has led health professionals to advise people to steer clear of potatoes, citing their supposedly high glycemic index. It's crucial to understand that blaming potatoes for blood sugar spikes is misplaced. If your blood sugar rises after consuming potatoes, it's not the fault of the potatoes; it's due to insulin resistance. To truly address this issue, you need to heal not just the insulin resistance but also your pancreas, kidneys, heart, damaged tissues, and more. It's a holistic approach that involves restoring your body's various systems. When you achieve this, your insulin sensitivity is restored, allowing you to enjoy potatoes in healthy preparations without causing spikes in your blood glucose levels. This signifies true healing and a life free from disease.

This potato misinformation has fueled the sugar versus fat versus protein debate, contributing to a crisis that's swiftly claiming lives. Do I want to silence those individuals that teach you to not eat potatoes if you suffer from insulin resistance?

No. We have a right to free speech. But I do want to help you—my readers—understand the science behind your chronic condition and ultimately put into practice what truly works to keep you chronic disease free and free of harmful medications and unnecessary medical appointments. We only have a set amount of time on this planet from the moment you are born to the moment you die—I want you to be able to use that time to realize your human potential in this lifetime. I want for you to live a life full of love, adventure, and joy in the myriad of ways that light you up. I want you to experience total health and life freedom.

Remember this one line in this book if can't remember anything else I've written:

"Avoiding wholesome and organic high-carbohydrate foods will not reverse or halt the progression of your diabetes; it may merely create more health problems. It gives a false sense of control over the disease, which ultimately harms your overall physical, mental, emotional, and spiritual health."

Navigate the Complexities of Nutrition with Ease

Eat Real to Heal empowers you with the knowledge and understanding to make informed, health-conscious choices independently. No more doubts, no more confusion. By the time you finish this book, you'll be equipped with the tools and insights to confidently decide what foods are best for your well-being. You'll gain a deep understanding of how to nourish your body, making those uncertainties about what's good or bad for you a thing of the past. This book will not only transform your relationship with food but also grant you the freedom to make choices that support your health without relying on anyone else's advice. Get ready to reclaim control over your nutrition journey and embrace a life of vibrant health and vitality.

The Science: There All Along

I've learned a lot more since I published this book in 2018. In fact, since then, an astonishing 68,000 studies have been published, all pointing to the remarkable benefits of a plant-based lifestyle, emphasizing nutrition as a powerful tool for preventing chronic diseases and highlighting the detrimental effects of harmful toxins. This surge in scientific evidence underscores a profound shift in our understanding of health. It's not merely a trend but a groundbreaking revelation that can revolutionize how we approach well-being.

This wealth of research signifies a pivotal moment in the way we view our health and the impact of our choices. The sheer volume of studies reflects a growing global awareness of the importance of nutrition and its role in preventing diseases that have plagued humanity for generations. It means we're not merely speculating; we're now armed with an arsenal of knowledge that proves the potency of whole, plant-based foods in promoting health and longevity.

Each study contributes to a growing body of evidence that validates the principles outlined in this book. It reinforces the idea that our bodies thrive on nutrient-dense, plant-based diets, and that by eliminating harmful toxins, we can create an internal environment conducive to healing. The significance of these studies lies not just in the data they present, but in the hope they offer. They provide concrete proof that our choices matter, that the foods we consume can either nourish or harm us, and that a shift toward a plant-based, toxin-free lifestyle is a scientifically substantiated path toward optimal health. This vast body of research empowers us to make informed decisions, supporting our journey toward a healthier, disease-free life.

Fire Your Doctor...

Is it time to consider a change in your healthcare approach? If your doctor isn't aware of the potential reversibility of chronic diseases, it might be a crucial moment to take action. You have two options: either educate your current doctor or fire your existing one. Or maybe just kindly part ways and seriously consider finding a healthcare provider who aligns with your beliefs about the reversibility of chronic conditions. In the wake of the COVID pandemic, it became evident that individuals with existing chronic diseases and high inflammatory markers were at significantly higher risk. This unfortunate reality became a catalyst for understanding the importance of building resilience in our bodies.

When facing the challenges posed by viruses and other environmental stressors, it is vital to reduce inflammatory markers, heal all organs and systems, and fortify our bodies against external threats. Our bodies are continually exposed to various environmental factors, including approximately eighty thousand unregulated toxic chemicals released into our surroundings annually. These substances, including those sprayed on our food and affecting our soil, hinder the growth of nutritious crops. A thought-provoking documentary, *The Need to Grow*, delves into this issue, shedding light on the critical connection between our environment and our health. www.theneedtogrow.com.

In light of these revelations, the emphasis on healing, resilience, and informed healthcare choices has never been more pressing. It's time to empower ourselves with knowledge, advocate for our well-being, and make decisions that support our bodies' ability to overcome challenges and thrive.

Going Beyond Common Sense

I can't help but share my frustration about the overwhelming abundance of health advice flooding our lives. It seems like every day there's a new book or a doctor unveiling yet another set of pillars, steps, or methods to reverse chronic diseases. But here's the thing—do we really need all these complicated strategies?

When will it become common sense that we should spend more time in nature, savor fiber-rich fruits and veggies, kick harmful habits like smoking and excessive drinking, practice the art of breathing, meditate, obtain a solid 8 hours of sleep, ensure our bowel movements are healthy and regular, and yes, move our bodies more? These aren't groundbreaking revelations; they're basic human principles grounded in simplicity and common sense.

And speaking of common sense, the World Health Organization (WHO) just confirmed what many of us already knew: there is no safe level of alcohol consumption for our health. I mean, it's not new information. Health coaches reading scientific studies have long been aware of the havoc alcohol can wreak on our bodies—just look at the countless lives and livers destroyed by this government-supported toxin.

So, let's cut through the noise and focus on what truly matters. We don't need more complexity, we need sincerity. It's about embracing the fundamental truths of well-being that often get lost in the maze of information. Fresh air, sunshine, greenery—nature provides some of the most potent healers. Fiber-packed fruits and vegetables, mindful living, and ample sleep are not just health tips; they're life essentials.

What we truly need is a mindset shift—a collective understanding of how to navigate our complex healthcare system. These twelve simple practices are not just recommendations; they are non-negotiables for a vibrant, healthy life. Let's make these practices not just a part of our routines but a part of our identities.

Reclaiming Your Health: Top 12 Tips for Lasting Empowerment and Healing

In the pursuit of reclaiming your health and seizing control of your life, knowledge becomes not just power but a guiding light. I am excited to share with you a transformative set of principles: the top twelve tips that will serve as your roadmap to wellness. These are not mere suggestions; they are tools of empowerment designed to help you regain mastery over your own well-being.

Number 1: Embrace the Power of Belief

The first fundamental principle is to understand and truly believe that your chronic condition is not an irreversible fate. It's a belief that can move mountains, for in acknowledging the potential for change, you unlock the door to your own healing. Your conviction becomes the bedrock upon which you rebuild your life and vitality, reminding you that your body is resilient, capable, and endlessly adaptable.

These tips are more than just steps; they are declarations of your agency, your power to heal, and your right to a vibrant life. By embracing these principles, you step into a future where your well-being is in your hands, where your health is a journey of empowerment, not a destination dictated by others. Let's embark on this transformative journey together, where your belief in the possibility of healing becomes the catalyst for profound, positive change.

Number 2: Persevere with Unwavering Determination

In your journey toward healing, persistence is your greatest ally. At Richer Health, we recognize that conventional treatments and medications can serve as essential crutches, especially when you are navigating uncharted territory on your path to reclaiming your health. There is no shame in relying on prescriptions or medical interventions while you gather the knowledge, build your support team, and chart your course toward optimal well-being.

Remember, this transformation takes time. It's a gradual process of learning, unlearning, detoxifying, and rebuilding—a process that unfolds step by step. Be patient with yourself. Know that healing is not a race but a deeply personal odyssey. We are here to support you every step of the way.

So, don't lose heart. Keep absorbing information, asking questions, and fostering belief in your body's capacity to heal. You are not alone on this journey; a community of support and knowledge surrounds you. By staying determined and steadfast, you are taking proactive steps toward a future where chronic diseases are not prison sentences but challenges you overcome. Keep going, and remember, every small effort is a monumental stride toward your renewed health and vitality.

Number 3: Cultivate a Dedicated Healthcare Team

In your pursuit of vibrant health, having the right support system can make all the difference. It's essential to assemble a healthcare team that is committed to delving deep into the roots of your health challenges. These professionals won't settle for quick fixes or superficial solutions; instead, they will diligently work alongside you until you are liberated from the shackles of your disease.

How will you know when you've truly triumphed? Your bloodwork, newfound freedom from symptoms, abundant energy, and the ability to embrace work with enthusiasm and vitality will be your undeniable signs of success.

But how do you go about forming such a team? We

understand this can be overwhelming, which is why we've created a comprehensive guide to help you assemble your Whole Health Team. This guide is designed to walk you through the process, ensuring you have the right individuals by your side, dedicated to unraveling the complexities of your health issues.

 To learn more and discover how to gather a team that will champion your well-being, click on this https://www.eatrealtoheal.ca/whole-health-team-exercise or scan the QR code. Armed with the right guidance, you can create a healthcare support network that empowers you on your journey to lasting health and vitality.

Number 4: Embrace the Power of Hyper Nutrition and Holistic Detoxification

In our fast-paced world, simply relying on regular nutrition may not be enough to combat the challenges of chronic diseases. Disturbingly, it's estimated that we have just sixty years of fertile soil left to cultivate our food. But fear not, there's a silent revolution happening beneath our feet, led by passionate individuals dedicated to revitalizing our soil. These unsung heroes are instrumental in ensuring our crops are nurtured in rich, nutrient-dense earth, allowing us access to food that can truly heal.

However, healing goes beyond just consuming food; it demands a targeted approach grounded in hyper nutrition. This approach involves embracing organic produce grown in biodynamic, soil-enriched environments. It incorporates the vitality of vegetable juicing, the potency of supplements, and the transformative power of daily liver detoxification, all intricately detailed in the pages of this book.

By adopting this holistic method, you open the pathways and channels within your body, paving the way for profound healing. This integrated approach, blending hyper nutrition with thorough detoxification, has been our guiding principle. It's how we've guided countless clients, even those once confined to hospital beds due to conditions such as chronic kidney disease, advanced arthritis, cystic fibrosis, unexplained weight loss from autoimmune disorders, and various other debilitating conditions, to reclaim their health and vitality.

By embracing this strategy, you, too, can embark on a transformative journey toward optimal health, breaking free from the clutches of chronic illness and reclaiming your life.

Number 5: Understand the True Definition of Reversing Chronic Diseases

In the pursuit of health, it's crucial to dispel a common misconception: there's no magic pill or quick fix capable of reversing chronic diseases. Beware of anyone promising a one-size-fits-all solution, for after years of experience, I can confidently affirm that such claims are misleading. Prescription medications, while sometimes necessary to manage symptoms temporarily, do not constitute a cure. They merely mask the signs of illness. Remove the medication, and the symptoms invariably resurface.

True reversal of a chronic disease paints a different picture. Picture this: savoring an array of nutrient-dense foods, including those rich in healthy carbohydrates, without fear of spiking blood sugar levels. Picture living medication-free, yet experiencing stable blood sugars, restored insulin sensitivity, vanquished disease symptoms, and boundless energy. Imagine a life where mental clarity reigns supreme, banishing the once-persistent brain fog. Envision a pain-free existence, absent of any painkillers, where your body feels truly alive.

This, my friend, is the essence of reversing a chronic disease. It's about reclaiming your vitality, embracing life without the burden of medications, and reveling in the joy of pain-free movement. Remember, true health is not found in the temporary alleviation of symptoms, but in the profound, lasting transformation of your entire being. Through dedicated efforts and holistic practices, you can achieve this reality, emerging stronger, healthier, and more vibrant than ever before.

Number 6: Embrace the Lifelong Journey to Wellness

A common question that often arises is, "How long do I need to follow this program?" Let me clarify: this is not a mere six-week endeavor that you undertake and then revert to your former lifestyle. The Eat Real to Heal program is designed as a transformative six-week transition into your new way of life. Within this timeframe, you'll learn the intricacies of preparing and consuming foods in a wholesome manner. You'll delve into the art of incorporating juicing, understanding the profound science behind its benefits in reversing chronic diseases.

In these six weeks, you'll unlearn the old narratives surrounding chronic diseases and supplements. It's a period for cleansing your cupboards, bidding farewell to processed and packaged foods that have contributed to your ailments. Restocking your shelves with the essential nine nutrients or supplements vital for supporting your journey towards chronic disease reversal is equally crucial.

Moreover, this transition phase allows you to gather your resources, educate your family and friends about your transformative journey, and master the delicate balance between art and science in the reversal of chronic diseases. Understanding the liver's pivotal role and learning the daily liver detox regimen are indispensable components of this phase.

By investing six weeks to craft this new lifestyle, you're essentially crafting a foundation for a lifetime of vibrant health. So, to answer the question of how long you should commit to this program: it's simple. You embark on this journey for as long as you desire to live a life unburdened by chronic diseases, ushering in an era of enduring wellness and vitality.

Number 7: Embrace Your Self-Worth

Recognizing your self-worth is not a swift realization but rather a lifelong practice, a journey that unfolds gradually. Often, my clients, especially women and those identifying as non-binary, display an innate tendency to prioritize the well-being of others over their own. It's not uncommon for them to approach me with the intention of learning this program to aid a loved one battling chronic illness, all while neglecting their own health issues.

In these instances, the paradox is stark: they harbor a wealth of knowledge and compassion for others but often disregard their own well-being. It's akin to pouring from an empty cup. This pattern, prevalent among many, leads to a near burnout state. Yet, healing oneself necessitates a fundamental shift—a profound understanding of your inherent worthiness. You must internalize that you are deserving of attention, time, and the deliberate creation of space in your life.

Imagine your life as an aircraft in turbulence; you are instructed to secure your own oxygen mask before assisting others. Likewise, your healing journey begins with self-care. By investing in your well-being, you become a living testament to the transformative power of healing. Only when you have nurtured your own health can you genuinely support others in their healing journey.

Let this knowing permeate your being, a knowing that you are worthy of the time and energy required to learn and implement the principles outlined in this book. Together, let's bolster each other in manifesting this awareness into practical, everyday practice, creating a community where self-worth is celebrated and upheld.

Number 8: Just Do It—Stop Procrastinating and Be Consistent

In the pursuit of transformation, there is no room for procrastination or excuses. The time for change is now. It's easy to delay, to convince ourselves that we will start after a particular event, a holiday, or a celebration. However, the essence of embracing a new lifestyle lies in your ability to prioritize your well-being consistently.

Picture this journey as a commitment—a covenant not just with yourself, but with the very Earth that nurtures you, the soil in which your food grows, and the future that awaits. To embark on this journey, you must place your body, mind, and health at the forefront of your priorities.

Shifting to a new lifestyle demands a steadfast commitment, a departure from the erratic patterns of yo-yo dieting and occasional cleanses. It calls for an unwavering dedication to values and principles that you embody every single day. Just as you consistently honor virtues like honesty, fidelity, nonjudgment, and truth, your approach to nutrition should mirror this steadfast commitment.

Consistency is the linchpin, the foundation upon which true wellness is built. By embracing this principle, you not only transform your life but also contribute to the health of generations yet unborn. Demand the best for yourself— opt for the healthiest, most nourishing foods, not only for your well-being but for the well-being of every generation that will follow. The power to create a healthier world lies within the daily choices you make. It starts now, with your unwavering commitment and consistent actions. So, just do it. Your future self will thank you.

Number 9: Be Discerning about the Nutrition Advice You Follow

It's crucial to seek guidance from practitioners who have successfully reversed chronic conditions in multiple clients. Don't hesitate to ask for proof of their track record. If a health practitioner claims confidentiality prevents them from connecting you with former clients, be cautious. Reputable professionals readily obtain patient consent for such discussions, allowing you to learn firsthand about the healing journey.

Additionally, avoid practitioners who treat you like a trial subject. If their approach involves experimenting with various methods without a clear plan, it might indicate a lack of expertise. Remember, your health deserves proven and reliable strategies, not guesswork.

Number 10: Demand Results and Timely Progress from Your Practitioner

It's essential to expect tangible results when addressing chronic conditions. In my experience, 99% of these issues can be reversed, often showing improvements within one to two weeks. Within three months, changes should be evident in your blood levels, urine tests, inflammatory markers, and symptomatology. If you don't see substantial progress, it's time to reconsider your therapy and seek a practitioner who delivers results instead of endless experimentation.

When I guide my clients, my aim is to empower them fully within a few hours, typically requiring only one or two follow-ups, which I provide without extra charges. My ultimate goal is their complete self-sufficiency—a state where they no longer require my assistance. Their family members often adopt the same principles, leading to a household free from chronic diseases. This outcome signifies effective healthcare.

Number 11: Challenge Discrimination in Disease Diagnosis

Refuse to accept discriminatory explanations for your health condition based on ethnicity, age, gender, or race. Such reasoning is a form of racism, sexism, and ageism. Genetic factors should only be considered if scientifically proven. As of this book's writing, the CDC lists factors like ethnicity, age, race, and gender as risk elements, but this is a misguided simplification. The genuine origin of most diseases lies in nutritional deficiencies and toxicity.

I firmly assert this truth from my extensive experience: once we address these core issues in my clients, they heal, regardless of their age, gender, or ethnicity. Discriminatory attitudes perpetuate ignorance and hinder our understanding of chronic illnesses. We must collectively raise our voices against this discrimination and advocate for a change in this narrative.

Number 12: Addressing Intergenerational Trauma for Holistic Healing

Acknowledging and confronting intergenerational trauma is pivotal in our healing journey. Trauma, whether suppressed or active, can profoundly impact our nervous system, making physical healing more challenging. Through the strategic use of food and detoxification, we build a resilient foundation, enabling profound spiritual, mental, and physical healing.

I've witnessed this transformative process repeatedly with my clients. As they follow the program outlined in this book, they find not only physical healing but also a deeper spiritual connection with themselves, others, nature, and the Creator. Our ultimate goal is holistic well-being: physical, spiritual, mental, and emotional health. However, focusing on physical health initially, by rebuilding a robust foundation and addressing nutritional deficiencies and toxicity, allows for a more efficient and graceful restoration of balance in the entire body.

Clients often report enhanced meditation experiences, and their physical ailments dissipate. By replenishing their bodies' energy, they overcome intergenerational trauma. Their increased mitochondrial energy, reduced physical pain, optimized brain function, restored microbiome, and balanced neurotransmitter levels lead to diminished anxiety and stress. This liberation from the burden of chronic diseases not only grants them physical relief but also frees up resources, both time and money, enabling them to invest in their emotional, spiritual, and mental well-being. This comprehensive healing approach fosters transformative change, propelling individuals toward a harmonious and balanced existence.

Our Shenanigans

Since the release of the first edition of *Eat Real to Heal*, our journey has taken an exhilarating turn.

Tony Robbins & *Eat Real to Heal*

We were deeply honored when Tony Robbins, a prominent figure in the world of personal development and wellness, recognized our work as a force for good. His endorsement led to a remarkable opportunity—being featured on his podcast, where he highlighted us as one of the top ten gifts of health. This recognition catapulted our message to a wider audience, opening doors to engagements that we could have only dreamed of.

One particularly memorable moment was when Tony Robbins and his platinum partners group visited Vancouver. We had the privilege of welcoming them at the airport, providing catering for their team, and forging connections that would prove to be invaluable. We were also invited onto Tony Robbins' podcast which was not just a validation of our efforts but a testament to the impact of our work.

During the podcast, I was honored to be acknowledged as a force for good and named one of his Top 10 Gifts of Health in 2019, a moment that reinforced our commitment to spreading the message of healing and well-being.

This recognition has fueled our dedication to the cause of holistic health and has motivated us to continuously refine and expand our offerings. As we move forward, our mission remains unwavering—to empower individuals with the knowledge and tools they need to reclaim their health, transform their lives, and contribute positively to the world around them. The journey from that initial edition to where we stand today is a testament to the power of perseverance, passion, and the profound impact that a single idea can have on the lives of many.

I'm a Doctor!

I'm incredibly excited to share some big news with you all—after seven mentally, emotionally, and physically tough years, I'm now officially a doctor! No, not the kind with a stethoscope and a prescription pad, but a doctor of social sciences. You might wonder, what does that mean for you, my cherished readers?

Imagine being an investigator, much like Inspector Gadget or Sherlock Holmes, but for social issues, health challenges, and the complexities of our world. My role is to dig deep, unravel the layers, and get to the root cause of your illnesses. I'm here to unearth the fundamental solutions that empower you to make the lifestyle changes needed to reverse chronic conditions.

Now, some people might debate the significance of a doctorate in social sciences. There's this misconception that being a "doctor" only applies to medical professionals. But let me assure you, my journey through social sciences has equipped me with a unique set of tools.

Being a social science researcher is akin to being a detective in a world filled with puzzles. I'm not just crunching numbers; I'm understanding motivations, societal structures, and the human experience. It's about delving into the intricacies of nutrition, deciphering the flaws in our medical system, and finding innovative solutions for our societies and our planet.

But why is social science research so valuable, you might ask? In the realm of our intricate world, where human behavior, beliefs, and cultures shape everything, understanding the social fabric is key. We deal with real people, real struggles, and real solutions. Our research isn't just about statistics; it's about stories, emotions, and the very essence of what makes us human.

When it comes to tackling issues like nutrition, healthcare disparities, and social injustices, social science research provides a holistic perspective. It embraces the qualitative aspects that hard sciences might miss—the narratives, the lived experiences, and the qualitative data that add depth to our understanding.

So, my dear readers, rest assured that my journey as a social science doctor means that I'm here to explore the depths of our challenges and illuminate the path toward solutions. Together, we will navigate the complexities of our world, uncover the truths about our health, and work towards a future where understanding and compassion reign supreme.

Since the publication of the first edition of *Eat Real to Heal*, my journey has taken me further into the realm of knowledge and academia. I am proud to announce the completion of my PhD, a significant milestone in my commitment to understanding and overcoming the challenges faced by Black, Indigenous, and People of Color

(BIPOC) communities in accessing the quality of foods essential for reversing chronic diseases. My dissertation focused on the intricate web of barriers that hinder BIPOC individuals from accessing nutritious foods, with a special emphasis on addressing the intergenerational trauma inflicted upon these communities since the dawn of colonization.

The research I conducted unveiled a staggering 736 distinct barriers that BIPOC individuals encounter, each of which has been meticulously identified, themed, and coded. One of the pivotal revelations from this study was that the obstacles to reversing chronic diseases extend far beyond mere food access; they are deeply intertwined with historical traumas and systemic injustices perpetuated through generations.

In light of these findings, I am thrilled to announce the forthcoming publication of a book titled *Rise Up*, a comprehensive summary of my research. This publication aims to shed light on the multifaceted challenges faced by BIPOC communities and serves as a call to action. I firmly believe that our society's health is contingent upon the well-being of its most vulnerable members. Currently, BIPOC individuals suffer from chronic diseases at rates four to eight times higher than their counterparts, highlighting the urgent need for systemic change.

To make this vital research accessible to all, I have ensured that it is not confined to academic circles. Instead, it is available in various formats, including a TED-like talk, a podcast series featured on our *Eat Real to Heal* podcast, a forthcoming journal article, and a succinct dissertation summary. My intention is to mobilize knowledge, empower communities, and spark conversations that drive meaningful change.

I invite you to explore my research, engage with its findings, and join me in amplifying these critical conversations. Together, we can dismantle barriers, advocate for justice, and foster a society where health and well-being are truly accessible to everyone. You can access my research at the following link: https://www.seatoskythrivers.com/ research-journey-nricherdocsocsci. Please share this invaluable resource with your family and friends, as every shared insight brings us one step closer to a healthier, more equitable world.

A New Kind of Medical Center

Since the release of the first edition of *Eat Real to Heal* in 2018, significant changes have unfolded in my journey and in the world around us. Our Richer Health Retreat Center, where individuals from diverse corners of the globe came together to learn and heal, has been transitioned, and we're currently in the process of dreaming, designing, and building a new one. Stay updated on our progress by visiting www.richerhealthretreatcenter.com.

Psychedelic Therapy

In my quest for understanding the profound potential of psychedelic therapy, I embarked on an extensive research journey, delving into the realms of altered states of consciousness and the therapeutic power they hold. Yet, my exploration didn't stop at scholarly pursuits; I personally embarked on transformative healing journeys, courageously diving deep into my own psyche. Through these experiences, I cultivated a profound sense of self-awareness, embracing the intricate tapestry of my own mind. The gifts that emerged from these ventures were plentiful: enhanced emotional intelligence, a newfound sense of empathy, and an expanded consciousness that allowed me to perceive the world in novel ways.

Guided by my passion for healing, I dedicated myself to becoming a psychedelic therapist, specializing in Internal

Family Systems therapy. This unique combination of rigorous research, personal introspection, and specialized training has equipped me with the tools to guide others on their own transformative journeys toward healing and self-discovery. In these intervening years, I did extensive research and underwent training to become a psychedelic therapist. The burgeoning research in the realm of psychedelic plant medicines has shown their profound efficacy in treating drug-resistant depression, mental health conditions, anxiety, PTSD, suicidal ideation, and trauma. To delve deeper into this transformative field, check out my upcoming book on psychedelic therapy for chronic disease healing and global wellness at www.kulandira.com.

Our Documentary

During this period, we also crafted the documentary *Grounded in My Roots*, a powerful exploration of my ancestral heritage in Malawi, Africa, and how I first discovered the healing potential of food as medicine. This documentary is a testament to the profound impact of reconnecting with my roots. You can watch it here at www.groundedinmyroots.com and please share it widely among your friends. Additionally, be sure to join the waitlist for my upcoming book, *Rise Up*, where I delve into this transformative journey.

Furthermore, our film *Food of Our Ancestors* is slated for release in 2025, following our ambitious twenty-two million-strong tour across Canada. As we eagerly anticipate its arrival, please enjoy our short documentary, *Grounded in My Roots*, and stay tuned for more updates on our upcoming projects.[3]

Rare Genetic Diseases

I want to share an incredible milestone in this ongoing

---

3 Watch our documentary here at www.groundedinmyroots.com.

journey—my willingness to work with clients dealing with rare genetic disorders. Initially, I hesitated, overwhelmed by the lack of information regarding the impact of nutrition and detoxification on these individuals. The scarcity of resources and mentors made me apprehensive. Yet, a brave woman approached me, seeking support for her battle against cystic fibrosis. She was forty years old, her body succumbing to the disease, landing her in the hospital fifteen times a year, each visit coupled with debilitating secondary infections and endless antibiotic treatments. Her life was governed by four hours of daily physical therapy, struggling to clear her body of stubborn mucus blocks.

Our objective was clear: we didn't aim to reverse her genetic condition; instead, we wanted to explore if our program could provide any relief. The results, nothing short of miraculous, have propelled Zoey into a thriving life. She now bravely combats common illnesses with her own immune system, no longer succumbing to relentless secondary infections. Each day is a testament to her strength and resilience, taking it one step at a time. Together, we navigate the uncharted territories of cystic fibrosis, unraveling the vital roles of nutrition and detoxification, especially in clearing the excessive mucus that plagues her body.

Zoey's journey, chronicled through our collaborative podcasts, serves as a beacon of hope. Through her firsthand experience with the Eat Real to Heal method, the world witnesses the transformative power of this approach. Stay tuned for our upcoming podcasts, where Zoey's experiences will shed light on this groundbreaking work, offering invaluable insights into the realm of rare genetic diseases and the potential for healing through the power of nutrition and detoxification.

The Age of Intuition Is Now

We are entering an era defined by intuition rather than sheer information. In this precarious time, while I vehemently oppose misinformation, I also reject the suppression of free speech under any form of dictatorial control. As of writing this book, it is vital to recognize that a staggering five hundred hours of YouTube content is uploaded every minute. We find ourselves submerged in the information age, drowning in a sea of data, making it nearly impossible for the average person to discern reality. That's why I advocate for transitioning into the age of intuition. To do this, we need a fundamental understanding of how our bodies and the Earth function, grounded in simple biological and chemical principles, which I can encapsulate in a few concise sentences.

We, as humans, are an integral part of nature; we are not superior to any rock, tree, bug, animal, body of water, molecule, or ounce of soil on this planet. In fact, we are dependent on all these elements in our environment because we are inseparable from it. We require nutrients and clean air, just like a houseplant does. We must keep our bodies free of toxins and eliminate waste daily, akin to our pets or animals found in nature. We crave love, respect, and attention, and in return, we must give love, respect, and attention to all living and sentient beings in nature. This mutual exchange, this reciprocity, is how indigenous peoples across the globe have lived throughout history. It forms the foundation of genuine sustainability, the essence of healing ourselves, healing our planet, and creating a future worthy of the next seven generations.

Embracing the age of intuition and healing demands unlearning much of what you've been taught about diets, chronic diseases, cleanses, calories, salt, fats, sugars, classifications of healthy eating, detoxing, potatoes, juicing, supplements, and more. Did you know there are over ninety thousand different supplements on the market, when our bodies require more than twenty-five thousand different nutrients? Our microbiome consists of over twenty-five thousand different bacteria, fungi, and parasites, the majority of which are beneficial. We must shift away from the reductionist mindset that seeks to control every aspect of our bodies and embrace a holistic approach. By providing our bodies daily with an abundance and diversity of high-quality nutrients, we build resilience naturally. From this foundation, our bodies will utilize what they need, eliminating the stress of calorie counting, weighing foods, and attempting to biohack our way to health.

You Can Do This

Reading this book might overwhelm you, evoke fear, or make you feel utterly exhausted contemplating the lifestyle changes needed. I urge you to take it slow. Breathe deeply. Maybe just read one line, one paragraph, or one chapter at a time. Take breaks, step outside, immerse yourself in nature, and reflect on what you've read, especially if you're listening to the audiobook. Then, encourage yourself to return and read the next chapter, and the next, one at a time. The magic lies in the actions you take daily to eliminate processed, refined, packaged, and harmful 'filler' foods from your diet. Instead, focus on consuming nutrient-dense foods grown sustainably. Supplement your diet with freshly made vegetable juices and supplements that provide missing nutrients not found in foods. Support your liver in its healing and detoxifying processes. This is where the transformative power of regenerative healing occurs, where chronic diseases dissolve, and where your path toward true health begins to unfold.

PART TWO:

Understanding—and
Beating—Chronic Disease

What Is a Chronic Disease?

A chronic disease is defined as a disease that lasts three months or more.

It's not a cold or flu that clears up within a few days. It's a disease that persists—causing long-term stress, pain, and frustration, reducing your quality of life, or even shortening your life.

Chronic diseases include arthritis, cardiovascular diseases such as heart attack and stroke, diabetes, autoimmune disorders, epilepsy and seizures, obesity, and cancer. Non-life-threatening conditions like acne, headaches, migraines, and skin conditions can be considered chronic disease, too. Anything that's happening in your body for a long time— several months in a row—that's a chronic disease.

Chronic diseases can be prevented, reversed, and eliminated—without medication.

How? By fueling yourself with real food, which repairs damaged cells, tissues, organelles, and organs, rebuilds your microbiome, boosts your immune system and metabolism, and allows your body to naturally fight disease effectively. That's what this entire book is about.

Why Do Chronic Diseases Happen?

After being diagnosed with cancer—or any other chronic disease—the first question that most people ask is, "Why?"

"Why is this happening to my body? Where does this disease come from? Is it genetic? Is it caused by toxins in the environment? Is it because I grew up next to a power plant that was always spewing smoke into the air? Is it because I used to drink Diet Coke every day? Is it caused by stress? Is it something I did, or didn't do? Did I exercise too much or too little? Is God punishing me or testing me?"

The answer is...

Maybe all of those things.

Maybe some of those things.

Maybe none of those things.

It's nearly impossible to know exactly why a chronic disease develops, because the causes can be "everything and anything."

So, if you've got cancer, what caused it? We don't know. We may never know.

In my opinion, the best course of action is to stop worrying about what happened in the past, and instead, take charge of your present and future.

Let's focus on what you can you start doing—right now, today—to boost your immune system and start healing.

Even though you may never know exactly why you got sick, the good news is that you have a great deal of control over your eating habits and lifestyle—and therefore, a great deal of control over your body's healing process.

Instead of obsessing about what caused your disease, let's focus on how to beat it.

Focus on what you're eating today. What you're drinking today. How you're taking care of yourself today.

Today can be the first day of a healthier, stronger, and, eventually, pain- and disease-free life.

Myths about Cancer and Other Chronic Diseases

Myth: Cancer is mostly caused by genetic factors.

This is false. Only 3–5 percent of chronic diseases, including cancer, are caused by genetic factors. The other 95 percent of chronic diseases are caused by a combination of non-genetic factors, including stress, lifestyle, eating habits, pollution, and many other environmental factors.

Even if you have a family history of cancer, this doesn't mean you're definitely going to get cancer, too. Epigenetic factors, the mechanisms other than your own DNA that switch genes on and off, can either promote healthy development or harm it. By upgrading your lifestyle—especially your eating habits—you can radically change your destiny.

Myth: The most effective treatment for cancer is chemotherapy.

This is false. Chemo has a very low success rate. For certain types of cancer, the success rate ranges from 2.1–42 percent. Can you imagine getting onto an airplane with a pilot who has a 2.1–42 percent success rate of landing the plane safely? It sounds insane, right? And yet, that's what we're doing when we put our bodies through chemo.

A recent poll asked doctors, "If you were diagnosed with cancer, would you choose chemo as your treatment?" 75 percent said no, because they're painfully aware of chemo's ineffectiveness.

Bottom line: chemo doesn't always work. In fact, it hurts more often than it helps. Chemo wreaks havoc on the body, weakening your immune system, making it more difficult to heal.

Should you say no to chemo? I can't make that choice for you. It's a deeply personal choice, and it's something that you and your health team must decide together. But, when making this life-altering decision, it's important that you have all the facts. To begin, ask your doctor, who should also be knowledgeable about nutrition, to help you understand how you could combine nutrition, chemotherapy, and other non-invasive treatments to increase your chances of healing for the long term.

Myth: Cancer is caused by viruses in the air.

This is false. Cancer is not caused by a virus. It's not something you can "catch" like the flu. However, there can sometimes be an indirect connection between viruses and cancer. When a virus enters the body, it may increase a person's risk of developing a certain type of cancer only because it first affects the body's immune system, not that the virus causes the actual cancer. Cancer begins in the body when a single healthy cell goes rogue, turns into a cancerous cell, is able to go undetected by the body, divides and multiplies either slowly or quickly over a period of time, and then, hopefully, gets caught before it's too late. When you're in a weakened state, you're more vulnerable to developing a chronic disease, such as cancer.

Myth: Toxins in the environment always lead to cancer.

Not exactly. Toxins are not good for us—that's obvious—but toxins impact different people's bodies in different ways.

For example, let's say your sister gets exposed to a harmful substance—fumes from a nearby power plant, for example—and she winds up getting cancer.

You grew up in the same household. You were exposed to that exact same substance for many years, too. But, instead of cancer, the toxicity might manifest in your body in a different way. It might manifest as multiple sclerosis,

Crohn's disease, eczema, allergies, psoriasis, or any number of chronic diseases. Or not at all.

So, when we are exposed to environmental stressors, it's not really possible to say who's going to get what. Sandra Steingraber's book *Living Downstream: An Ecologist's Personal Investigation of Cancer and the Environment* is a brilliant account of the link between cancer and exposure to environmental pollutants.

Myth: Some people are just born with bad DNA. They're born with bad cells that are cancerous.

This is not accurate. Cancer starts from one single cell or small group of cells—cells that were, at some point, healthy cells.

Sometimes, for a whole variety of reasons—environmental and physical stressors, toxicity, nutritional deficiency, immune system suppression, hormonal imbalances—that one single cell becomes mutated.

When a cell becomes mutated, we have all kinds of defenses in our bodies that immediately go onto high alert. They want to detect that mutated cell and kill it, destabilize it, gobble it up, and spit it out. Hooray! This is your immune system working optimally and doing its job.

Sometimes, though, for all kinds of reasons, your body doesn't catch that mutated cell in time. That mutated cell is left to its own devices. It can then divide and grow in an uncontrolled way. It eventually grows and grows and grows until it becomes a tumor. That's how cancer starts: One cell mutates, starts to grow exponentially, and then takes over the body.

But that one cell started from a healthy cell. So, the question is, how can we keep all of our cells healthy? How can we keep our immune system beautifully active? One answer, of course, is to upgrade the food we put into our bodies—by eating real food, every day.

Myth: Cancer is caused by bad karma.

Absolutely not. There are plenty of kind, compassionate people who get cancer, and there are plenty of cruel, vicious people who don't get cancer. Cancer is not caused by evil thoughts and deeds, or "bad karma," as it's sometimes called.

That being said, there is a connection between your mindset and your physical body.

Numerous studies confirm that creating a positive mindset can accelerate the healing process. If you spend three minutes meditating each morning, or writing down three things you feel grateful for, or simply breathing deeply, hugging someone for a minimum of twenty seconds, or listening to an uplifting song that you love, these small actions will decrease your stress levels and increase the healing capacity of your body.

Decreased stress means decreased levels of cortisol (the stress hormone). Lower cortisol means your body can function optimally and heal faster.

To be clear, I'm not saying, "Think positive thoughts and your cancer will disappear." That's an unrealistic statement, especially if you are the one of many who also suffer from "monkey-mind" or an unsettled or indecisive mind. But, if you cultivate an optimistic, positive mindset, it will support your healing process. Without a doubt, a positive mindset is more beneficial than a negative one.

In the fight against disease, you want to give yourself every possible advantage—and that includes boosting your mood with positive thoughts and reducing stress every way you possibly can.

Myth: Switching to real food will cure cancer, every time.

I wish this was true. It's not. Switching to real food is a powerful choice, a choice that will strengthen your body, boost your microbiome, which will in turn boost your immune system, and give you the best possible chance at making a full recovery. But it's just that—*a* chance. Not a 100-percent guarantee.

I've seen hundreds of patients beat their cancer, and other chronic diseases, by following the guidelines in this book. But it does not work every single time.

Just this last year, a young girl was slowly dying in a hospital when her parents called me in for a health consult. She was battling a terminal form of cancer and the doctors said that chemotherapy, surgery, and radiation wouldn't help her. Her parents wanted to give her every possible chance at surviving. We collaborated with this girl's doctors and nurses, and we put her on a nutrition and detox plan with the highest-quality food that money can buy. The day I arrived, the hospital kitchen was serving every child on the oncology ward hotdogs on refined white flour buns, chocolate pudding, cow's milk, and such a small sprout of raw broccoli that I barely noticed it on the plate. Fortunately, my young client wouldn't touch this cancer-causing food. We placed this girl on an organic, clean, nutrient-dense program. We flooded her body with nourishment. The nurses helped her detoxify her body safely. We gave her body every possible advantage. But, in the end, it wasn't enough.

Prior to being hospitalized with stage IV cancer, her doctors had misdiagnosed her for months, sending her home with a Metamucil and pain medication treatment plan, before realizing that she actually had cancer. She did outlive her medical team's prognosis by a few months—she had been given three weeks to live—but she eventually passed away, months later, at home, in her parents' grieving arms.

What the diet change had done was to boost her levels high enough to allow her to be released from the hospital, to go home to play with her siblings, parents, and horses. Prior to starting the therapy, her medical team had said she would never be able to leave the hospital, and that she would die there, in her hospital bed. Only if the nutritional therapy could improve her lab results would she be allowed to go home and live out the rest of her life among loved ones in the comfort of her familiar surroundings. I grieved with her parents, and still grieve her loss today, as I wonder what would have happened if the doctors hadn't misdiagnosed her for months on end, and if she could have started the therapy when her first symptoms appeared.

Sometimes, cancer steals people away, no matter how hard we try to beat it. It's unfair. But it happens.

With diseases, we need to be frank, honest, and realistic. There are no miracle cures. There's nothing—no pill, no chemo regime, no eating plan—that has a 100 percent success rate. We can't guarantee success. But we can boost the likelihood of success by eating real, whole, unrefined foods (not processed junk), resting, gently exercising, avoiding toxins (cigarette smoke, chemical-laden beauty products, excessive alcohol), and shifting stress. These lifestyle choices make a huge difference.

What Is the Gerson Therapy?

Throughout this book, you'll see me mention something called the Gerson Therapy.

What is Gerson Therapy? It's a form of nutritional therapy (basically, a "way of eating") that's designed to nourish and detoxify your body and restore it, so it can do what it's innately designed to do—heal itself. To reverse disease, the Gerson protocol is the ideal way to eat.

Right now, there are only two hospitals in the world that

offer the Gerson Therapy, though there are countless centers that have integrated its nutrition and detox plan into their kitchens and protocols. One is located in Mexico. The other is in Hungary. Why only two? The reasons for this are...very complicated.

When it comes to cancer, physicians in North America are legally obligated to recommend chemo, surgery, radiation, or sometimes gene therapy or immunotherapy.

Physicians are not allowed to recommend nutrition-based therapies to heal cancer or any other chronic disease. Physicians have to recommend something that has gone through an FDA clinical trial, like a pill, an injection, or a chemical treatment like chemotherapy.

That's why you'll never find a US or Canadian doctor recommending that you try the Gerson Therapy. If they prescribed it, they'd be at risk for losing their license.

Why Hasn't the Gerson Therapy Been FDA-Approved?

You might be wondering, "Why hasn't the Gerson Therapy gone through an FDA trial? If it's so effective, why hasn't it been FDA-approved so that physicians can prescribe it?"

There are numerous complex reasons, but the primary reason is lack of funding.

One clinical study can cost $50 million or more. Pharmaceutical companies can cough up this kind of money, no problem, and they do so repeatedly.

But people who work in the field of alternative healthcare— people who encourage patients to eat apples, collard greens, and carrots, like me? Sadly, funders who can write $50 million checks aren't exactly lining up around the block to fund research on organic produce. They'd never make their money back like they would from the billions of dollars in pharmaceutical prescription sales. We need a complete system overhaul when it comes to how we perform and fund randomized controlled trials.

Another reason is that the Gerson Therapy is complex, right? And science doesn't like complex. It wants to be able to measure everything. Think of the hundreds of macro variables within the Gerson Therapy that would be part of a clinical trial: the different fruits, vegetables, grains, legumes, spices, supplements, stress relievers like meditation, Qigong, yoga, sleep, coffee enema, juices, cooked versus raw foods, and more. Then dive deeper and consider the micro-variables within the Gerson Therapy. Researchers would never be able to know what reversed your disease or caused healing because of the diversity of micro-variables—the amino acids, enzymes, proteins, fats, sugars, molecules, atoms, ahhhhhh—it's just toooooo complicated for researchers to grasp, and therefore they don't want to or can't engage in these types of studies. However, with creative thinking, clinical trials could be designed to study the effectiveness of the Gerson Therapy for many different types of chronic degenerative illnesses. But until that happens, are you going to wait around for science to catch up and tell you that it is effective, or will you simply pull out your juicer and kitchenware and prove it for yourself?

Until science does catch up, we are stuck with a situation that's not ideal. We know the Gerson Therapy works, but there's no funding to get it FDA-approved, so doctors' hands are tied. Legally, doctors can't recommend Gerson, even if they want to (and many of them do). Patients have to seek it out on their own.

The pessimistic part of me believes that pharmaceutical companies don't ever want nutrition-focused treatments like Gerson to be FDA-approved because there's no financial benefit in it for them.

It's similar to how most oil companies haven't supported clean, renewable energy—in fact, they worked hard to oppose it. Oil, coal, and other fossil fuel companies constantly flex their big muscles, budgets, and governmental influence to block bills that would constrict their sales. They don't want clean energy to thrive, because that would be bad news for their industry. They want to crush clean energy options and continue to dominate the marketplace. But that's until the collective masses and innovative visionary companies like Tesla start demanding these sustainable changes.

Perhaps my perspective is overly pessimistic. Perhaps pharmaceutical companies really do have the best of intentions. Perhaps they really care about helping sick people to get well. Perhaps. But, as the saying goes, "Follow the money." If pharma companies had a financial incentive to secure FDA approval for non-toxic, non-chemical treatments like the Gerson Therapy, I bet it would have happened already.

To be clear, I have the utmost respect for the medical profession. We need surgeons. We need nurses. We need X-ray technicians. We need this entire industry. I'm definitely heading to the emergency room if I have a rock climbing accident or I find myself in a car crash or one of my daughters contracts an infectious life-threatening illness.

But, as patients, we can't go into the doctor's office and blindly follow their guidance, because they don't always have all the answers. And sometimes, doctors are actually prohibited from recommending a course of action that, deep down, they wish they could recommend.

Remember this. Just because a doctor prescribes a pill, antibiotic, injection, chemo, or radiation, that doesn't mean it's actually the best option for you. It just means it's what they're "obligated" to recommend to you.

The History of the Gerson Therapy

The history of the Gerson Therapy is fascinating. It all started with Max Gerson, MD, back in the 1910s, when he was still a relatively new doctor.

As a young man, Gerson suffered from terrible migraines. Often, the pain was so intense, he couldn't meet with patients. He spent hours vomiting and had to lie down in a dark room. It was debilitating. He was desperate to find a cure.

One day, Gerson found some literature that suggested that changing your diet could reduce pain and improve your health. He didn't know anything about this, because he never studied nutrition in medical school. He'd been taught how to diagnose diseases, how to disinfect a wound, how to set a broken bone, how to perform a surgery. But using food as a form of healing medicine? That was never covered in med school.

Being a researcher and a scientist, Gerson felt curious about this paper he'd read. Could it be true? He figured it couldn't hurt to try and see.

Using his body as a living laboratory, he did a series of experiments. He began by eating large quantities of different types of foods to see if they would trigger a migraine or not. He did this with all types of food: high doses of meat, of salt, of vegetables, and so on. He experimented with processed and unprocessed foods.

He quickly realized that eating plant-based foods—ideally, fruits and vegetables straight from the garden—eliminated his migraines entirely. Other foods? Not so much.
For example, he could eat baskets of apples and never trigger a migraine—but if he ate a big portion of food that was canned and preserved in salt, or large portions of meat, it would trigger a migraine.

This is how Gerson began to define what he called "desirable foods" and "non-desirable foods." He devoted the rest of his life to studying the connection between food and disease.

Over the years, Gerson performed autopsies to examine the bodies of people who'd died from many chronic diseases, including cancer. Through these autopsies, he noticed two factors: a buildup of toxicity, and nutritional deficiency.

He began to wonder, "What if we could fix these two issues—remove toxicity and replenish nutrient deficiencies—using food as a form of medicine?"

He began a series of experiments, flooding patients' bodies with nutrient-dense food and juices. The results were remarkable. Tumors shrank. Women who struggled with infertility were able to get pregnant. Terminally ill cancer patients recovered and lived an additional twenty, thirty, even forty years. This research became the foundation of what's now called the Gerson Therapy.

From Death's Door...Back to Life

One of the most famous Gerson experiments was conducted by Gerson and his colleague, Dr. Ferdinand Sauerbruch. Together, they ran a clinical trial on tuberculosis, which, at the time, was considered an incurable disease.

Dr. Sauerbruch describes this famous clinical trial in great detail in his autobiography, "Das War Mein Leben". He gave Dr. Max Gerson a tuberculosis ward with 450 end-stage TB patients and told him that if he could cure even just one patient, he would believe everything that Gerson claimed about this plant-strong therapy. After several weeks, results were not noticeable and therefore Sauerbruch wrote Gerson to cancel the experiment, which was deemed a total failure. However, after posting the letter,

Sauerbruch discovered that one of his nurses was sneaking an assembly of the processed and refined 'treats' to the patients when Sauerbruch was not present. Sauerbruch later fired the nurse and assigned guards on the doors of the ward, and saw to it that the patients got the full Gerson Therapy. The trial continued and of the 450 patients with tuberculosis, 446 or 99% of the "incurable" cases were cured in the first clinical trial of Gerson's therapy. If that sneaky nurse had not been caught, the trial would have stopped and these results would never have been realized.

Sadly, I can relate to this story. I've met people newly diagnosed with cancer or another life-threatening disease, and had them tell me in June, "I'm sick, so I want to have a fun summer and really enjoy myself. I want to live life to the fullest and have all my favorite things." They spend the summer eating cheeseburgers, fries, and milkshakes, drinking beer, and having a big steak every other night, and then by September...they were dead.

I can't help but wonder, "Could we have reversed their disease if they'd been willing to make some changes?" It's impossible to know for certain, but the answer is, "Potentially, yes." And now we'll never know, because they're gone. It breaks my heart.

This is why I am relentlessly passionate about helping people upgrade their eating habits—because, oftentimes, it can mean the difference between life and death.

I wish more people would choose real food—clean, organic, plant-based food—but of course, I can't force anybody to do this. We all have to make this choice individually. You can choose to give yourself the best possible fuel, or, like those nurses who worked for Dr. Gerson, you can decide that it's more "fun" to eat garbage and harm your body. Personally, that doesn't sound like "fun" to me, but, ultimately, the choice is yours.

And I've been where you are today, wondering if the effort to clean up my diet or the pain of letting go of those addictive foods was worth it. Years ago, while building my businesses, I burned myself out. I was eating out every day, and, though I was choosing the healthiest vegetarian options that cafes and restaurants offered at that time, the foods I was consuming were still not organic—they were full of cell-damaging glyphosate and overloaded with refined flours, sugar, salt, and oils. I was consuming cell-damaging meals and was simultaneously highly stressed, constipated, and not sleeping: a perfect recipe for a health disaster.

My lab results proved it. What prompted me to head to the doctors and start collecting my baseline health data was that my joints ached worse than those of a ninety-year-old with lifetime arthritis, my heart was experiencing palpitations and misfires, my skin was so sensitive and painful that I couldn't even enjoy a light-touch massage, I suffered from insomnia, I had no libido, my teeth hurt, my brain felt like it was in a constant fog, and I couldn't concentrate or complete a task. My body was experiencing severe inflammation, and my blood work showed this to be true. My ESR and CRP levels were through the roof. My doctor, a highly intelligent integrated-health-care medical doctor, a loving mother of two, and someone who knew about my hectic lifestyle, put my file down, placed her hands on my shoulders, looked me sternly in the eyes and told me point-blank, "If you don't start practicing what you preach, you are going to have a heart attack in less than five years." Knowing that I wouldn't accept prescription drugs, she gave me a dose of my own medicine: "Stop everything you are doing right now and start doing the Gerson Therapy."

My MD's care, attention, and frankness provided the kick in the behind that I needed. My poor lab results, coupled with my severe symptoms, served as the reality check that I needed. As a mother of three beautiful girls, I knew that I could no longer play the martyr. I needed to heal myself now or suffer the consequences later, which wasn't an option. So, I called everyone I knew, my staff, my husband, my family and friends, and I told them that I would be out of commission for the next month, or until I healed myself.

I started the Gerson Therapy that day, and within three days, my skin pain was gone. My teeth no longer hurt. Within five days, my joints no longer ached. I can't recall how long it took for my heart palpitations to stop, but it was definitely less than two weeks, as that's when I had my next set of lab work completed and my inflammatory markers were back to normal. Yes—it took less than two weeks! I had lived with these symptoms for nearly two years. By the end of the month, all my symptoms had disappeared. I was pooping like a queen and sleeping like a baby. Libido?—Yes, ma'am!

This wasn't surprising to me, as I've had thousands of clients over the last decade who all had similar healing stories, no matter what their diagnosis or disease was. I was, however, grateful to my body for healing itself, and to myself for not waiting a second longer to get started.

And you can too.

Become the CEO of your own health. Simply copy what Kris Carr of *Crazy Sexy Cancer* did in her journey to heal herself. She became the CEO of a company that she dubbed "Save My Ass Technologies, Inc."

As Phil Knight, CEO of Nike, says: "Just do it."

The Six Components of Gerson Therapy

There are six components to the Gerson Therapy. For best results, all of them need to be practiced together. The six components are:

1. **Juicing** to reverse nutrient deficiency. (Think of it as an IV transfusion of nutrients and enzymes directly into your bloodstream, requiring no valuable digestive energy because the fiber is removed... and don't worry, you'll be getting plenty of fibre on this program through the three meals a day you are required to eat.)

2. **Eating real whole, unprocessed, unrefined food,** also to reverse nutrient deficiencies, plus it provides your body and microbiome with the much-needed plant-based insoluble fiber that you can't get anywhere else.

3. **Detoxifying the liver** through coffee enemas. (If your eyes are bulging in terror, stay calm. We'll discuss this later in the book. It's not as terrifying as you might think, and the science behind this fabulous liver detox is what makes it so effective at helping your body to heal and reverse disease.)

4. **Taking supplements** to replenish the body with nutrients that can't be absorbed from food alone, and to help your body digest your food and juices so that you can acquire even more nutrients from every morsel.

5. **Rest.** It's crucial to conserve energy for healing, especially when you're dealing with a life-threatening condition.

6. **Exercise.** Now, this may surprise you, but exercise is limited to activities like yoga, Qigong, gentle walking, etc., in this program, until you are fully healed, your symptoms are completely gone, and your illness doesn't stand a chance of returning.

People often ask, "Do I really need to do all six? Is that totally necessary?"

If you want to pick just one or two to do such as the food and rest, that's fine, and it's definitely better than nothing at all. You will notice improvements. But, for best results, I recommend that you practice **all six components for five weeks in a row**. After five weeks, you may pass up the supplements or increase the amount of exercise you do, if you wish (I can feel you exhaling a sigh of relief already!), but you'll want to keep the other components going. But, remember, this isn't a diet, it's a lifestyle change—so consider sticking to all six components for the full five weeks, just to experience the true self-healing power of your body. Don't be surprised if you want to continue this program forever!

Before you read further, ask yourself these questions regarding each of the six components:

1. **Juicing:** Why wouldn't I want to take extra nutrients into my body each day using the easiest method possible? (Think Ensure, but healthy.) After all, an apple today contains 80 percent less nutrients than it did twenty years ago, as so much of our food is grown in nutrient-deficient soil. And for those of you who have kids and can't get them to eat their veggies, juicing is a great way to make sure they are getting their nutrients.

2. **Real Food:** Do I really want to put foreign, addictive chemicals in my body and on my family's kitchen table that are known to cause cancer and create chronic disease, when I know that there are over three hundred thousand foods on this planet that are designed to keep my body free of cancer and disease?

3. **Liver Detox:** Knowing that each year, industries and government dump over eighty thousand poorly-monitored toxic chemicals into our air, land, water, cleaning, cosmetic, and food systems each year,

why wouldn't I want to support my liver with coffee enemas to flush those toxins out daily or weekly?

4. **Supplements**: Before I pose the question, you'll need some background data.

    a. **Point 1**: Prescription medications kill more North Americans each year than illegal drugs (just over a hundred thousand people, according to the Centers for Disease Control and Prevention, or CDC).

    b. **Point 2**: The CDC evaluated the safety of dietary supplements in a long-term study which found that, not only did no one die in the ten-year study period, but there was also not one adverse event reported from the use of dietary supplements.

    c. **Point 3**: Lastly, as I mentioned earlier, produce today contains nearly 80 percent less nutrients than it did twenty years ago, due to the fact that industrial farmers only put three nutrients back into depleted fields: PKN, or phosphorus, potassium, and nitrogen, when soils and produce require more than eighty-two different nutrients to be considered truly healthy.

So, knowing these three points, here's the question that you need to ask yourself: Why wouldn't I take nutritional supplements to replenish my nutritional deficiencies and give my body the best chance at repairing itself?

5. **Rest**: I know that the body needs rest when it's injured or ill, and everyone knows that eight solid hours of sleep a night, after a normal day of work or life, is a requirement, so why would I compromise my health by sacrificing my rest time?

6. **Exercise**: Wouldn't it be a good idea to conserve my

energy for repairing and regenerating my body, so that I'll actually have a vital body full of unlimited energy, and ensure that I can do all the exercise my strong heart desires for as long as possible?

We'll discuss all six components in more detail throughout this book.

And if your head is already spinning with too much information, please know this...the Gerson Therapy is, essentially, just a quick way of saying, *eat real food, detox daily, and take good care of your body.* It's not complicated. In fact, once you've transitioned into this lifestyle, you'll find that it's really simple to maintain.

Frequently Asked Questions about Food and Disease

Let's imagine we're sitting down together on a comfy couch. You've probably got several questions at this point, right? Let's have a glass of fresh, tasty carrot juice and talk through a few things that might be on your mind.

Question: I know it's better to eat organic food. But how important is it, really?

It's REALLY important. All caps. Non-negotiable. I can't emphasize this enough.

Our goal is to remove toxins from your body, and that's virtually impossible if you're eating strawberries that have been saturated with pesticides, particularly the herbicide glyphosate. I urge you to make organic food a top priority.

There's a popular conception that organic food is more expensive, but that's not always true. If you visit the local farmer's market, you can often find organic produce that's cheaper than non-organic produce at your neighborhood grocery store. If you're pressed for time, you can get it delivered! In many cities, you can get a lovely, bountiful box of organic produce delivered to your home or office. Google "Farm Box" or "CSA Box" (it stands for "Community-Supported Agriculture") to see the options in your area.

Also, Google "Sherry Strong." She's a wonderful friend of mine, and she has a wonderful program called "How to eat organic for $70 a week or less." Check it out. Make this happen for yourself. Your body is worth it.

Question: I've seen blogs and books that recommend eating raw food rather than cooked food. Is that a good idea? Shouldn't I go raw?

Raw, uncooked food—in moderation—can be great. But not 100 percent of the time.

Heat is our friend. Cooked food is our friend. Raw food is our friend, too. But too much raw food can be really tough on an already weakened digestive system. Often, it's more difficult to absorb nutrients from food that's totally raw, unless it's juiced, so if you're doing a totally raw diet, your body might be struggling to use more energy to break down and absorb everything it needs. Also, the long-term consumption of foods high in oxalic acid, which gets broken down by heat, can lead to nutrient deficiencies. This can throw your body seriously out of whack—even worse, could lead to a chronic degenerative disease. When you eat foods that are heated, such as cooked spinach, broccoli, Brussels sprouts, and others, you will absorb higher levels of vitamins, amino acids (which turn into protein in the body), fiber, and other macronutrients. These nutrients also become more absorbable. As with all vegetables, there are pros and cons to eating both raw and cooked forms of food. I suggest eating a wide array of fresh, whole plant foods in both raw and cooked form. This will provide you with the richest array of nutrients.

I'll never forget one Green Moustache customer who proudly told me that he was switching to a raw-food diet. I was skeptical and encouraged him to reconsider. But he was adamant. A few months later, he found himself in the hospital with severe stomach pain, digestive issues, and his weight had dropped to ninety-seven pounds on a six-foot frame. After switching back to a raw/cooked combo, his health returned. Let this be a cautionary tale. Know that, if you are already suffering from a chronic illness, jumping into a raw-food regime too quickly and without the right knowledge or coaching may set your health back even further. Enjoy a combination of cooked food and raw food. Both. Not just one or the other.

Question: You recommend drinking juice. Can I have a smoothie instead?

Smoothies are great. I love a great-greens, fresh-squeezed orange juice, and banana smoothie. Yum! But when it comes to flooding your body with nutrients, juicing is the best way to go. This is because juicing extracts all the nutrients from veggies and fruits, but without the bulky fiber. This allows you to consume more cold-pressed juice each day, which means you consume more minerals, vitamins, and other nutrients each day, which means you restore your nutritional deficiencies faster and with less digestive stress.

Imagine a glass of green juice or a glass of carrot-apple juice. You can take a few pounds of organic produce and distill it into an eight-ounce glass of juice. That single glass is packed with tons of vitamins and minerals, tons of nutrients that your body will love and desperately need. It's highly concentrated liquid medicine. Again, think of IV fluids tapping directly into your blood stream.

To get those same nutrients in a smoothie form or by eating them individually, you'd probably need to drink a sixty-four-ounce smoothie, because smoothies are much bulkier than juice, and they're filled with more air, water, and veggie and fruit fibre, which misses the entire point when it comes to juicing. That's why I recommend juicing rather than making smoothies. Basically, juicing is a more efficient way of delivering nutrients to your body.

If you don't have a juicer, there are several models that range from $49 to $349. The top-notch juicers are $1,000 and above. If that sounds like a lot of money, consider the daily breakdown. If you get a $1,000 juicer and you use it every day for one year, that's about $2.75 a day. Now, compare that to a $6.50 Starbucks latte that you drink once and it's gone forever—minus the toxins, dyes and sugar overload left behind! With a juicer, the per-use cost is low. It's an affordable luxury, and—unlike that Pumpkin Spice Latte that's packed with refined sugar and chemicals I can't even pronounce—juicing is a gift for your body.

Tip: Given that people have been juicing for hundreds of years, consider buying a used juicer off of Craigslist, Kijiji, or another site, and you'll save hundreds of dollars.

Question: I struggle with intense cravings. Some days, I just NEED a chocolate chip cookie or a cheeseburger. How can I give up my favorite foods?

Most North Americans are accustomed to eating lots of processed, heavily salted, sugared, and oily food, and lots of dairy, grain, and meat. In most households, that's how we are raised, so that's what we're familiar with, and that's what we crave. Actually, it's what your microbiome craves.

What's interesting, though, is that after switching to real food for a couple of weeks, your taste buds regenerate, your entire gut flora is replaced in just six days, and, therefore, your preferences begin to shift. You'll find yourself craving different things—like butternut squash soup, or collard green wraps stuffed with yam, potato, and shredded beets, or a nice glass of carrot-apple juice, or a big, comforting bowl of Hippocrates Soup. You can fill your day with delicious, tasty food—it's just going to be clean, nutrient-dense food instead of the junky disease-causing version.

Most of my clients never go back to the way they used to eat. Some will incorporate minimal amounts of organic meat and eggs into their routine on special occasions, but very few people go completely back to their previous way of eating. They feel so much better...so they don't want to!

Trust that this shift will happen for you, too. It might take a few days or weeks, but at a certain point, you will realize, "Wow. I feel amazing. I love eating this way. It's not a 'chore' to maintain this new lifestyle. It's a joy."

Question: But I love salt and food just doesn't taste good without it. Plus, isn't salt good for you?

It's true—you won't be using sodium salt during this five-week *Eat Real to Heal* program. In fact, you can go ahead and throw away your salt shaker(s) for good. Yes, just about every system in your body needs salt to make if function well; however, not all salts are created equal, and they are made up of a diversity of minerals.

What most people think of as "salt" is actually an aggressive substance called sodium chloride. Most processed foods contain high quantities of this substance for a variety of reasons, but primarily for food preservation—so it can last on a shelf indefinitely. The consequence of consuming sodium chloride is that it creates a highly acidic environment in your body, causing your cells and tissues to store excess water to neutralize the salt.

Mother Nature has designed our food brilliantly, keeping sodium salt to a minimum within our plant-based foods and keeping the beneficial, health-promoting "salts"—minerals like potassium, magnesium, calcium, and others—in abundance. If you consume a vibrant and abundant variety of plant-based whole foods, you'll never have to worry about being "salt" deficient. Excessive consumption of sodium salt can lead to uric acid buildup, cellulite, arthritis, gout, kidney stones, gallstones, cardiovascular disease and severe, irreparable tissue-damage syndrome.

The Gerson Therapy and the Eat Real to Heal program will provide you with all of the good "salts" while naturally eliminating the bad "salts," which will in turn regulate salt metabolism, which will restore your body's natural self-healing and repair mechanisms.

PART THREE:
Your New Lifestyle Begins

Ready to Reverse Disease and Feel Amazing?

Hopefully, by now, you're feeling inspired to upgrade your eating habits and begin a beautiful new chapter in your life.

You're ready for... More energy. Less pain. Less inflammation. Clear skin. Strong nails and hair. A powerful immune system that's operating at peak capacity. A solid chance at preventing and reversing chronic diseases, including cancer.

You can already see the innumerable rewards and benefits that are waiting for you...and you're ready to take the plunge.

Do you hear that? I'm sitting in my office, and I'm clapping and cheering for you! Yesss! Let's begin!

When I work with clients in person, at retreats, and in my online programs, I typically encourage people to begin with a "five-week challenge."

Follow the *Eat Real to Heal* guidelines for five weeks in a row and not only see how you feel, but also witness the physical changes that will occur.

For most people, five weeks feels like a manageable, not-too-scary commitment. It's not an eternity, but it's long enough to see some impressive changes.

However, it's important to remember that this isn't a "five-week diet." It's a new lifestyle, not a temporary blip.

Consider this:

Would you ever say to your child, "Sweetheart, I want you to be a kind, compassionate person for five weeks—and after that, you can be a jerk and be cruel to everyone"?

No! Obviously, you'd never say that. You want your child to be a kind person all the time, always and forever, not just for five weeks.

It's the same when it comes to your health. You're not going to take good care of your body for five weeks and then stop. You're going to continue. You're making a permanent lifestyle change—a change that comes with so many rewards.

Testimonial

I had twenty-two random guests join the first five-week challenge that I ever delivered. I offered it in person and based it out of our Green Moustache location in Whistler, British Columbia, Canada. Each week, I'd teach these twenty-two inquisitive students how to actually use food as medicine. During the wrap-up potluck at the end of the five weeks, one student, Sharon, shared her healing story with our group. Before starting the five-week *Eat Real to Heal* challenge, Sharon, a thirty-three-year-old woman, had found that she couldn't get pregnant because of a rare autoimmune disorder. Her endocrinologist scheduled her for a thyroidectomy, or surgery to remove her thyroid gland, followed by radiation and medication. Instead, Sharon delayed her surgery and did our program for the full five weeks. Much to her endocrinologist's surprise, her new lab results and doctor's visit revealed that Sharon had eliminated her symptoms, repaired her thyroid, and rebalanced her hormones and other blood levels. I'm pleased to announce that she also gave birth to a beautiful bouncy baby boy less than one year later and has been symptom-free since. Sharon still follows the principles of the five-week program, of course.

The Best Time to Change Your Lifestyle Was Yesterday

The Second-Best Time Is Today

In this section of the book, we'll cover what to eat (meal ideas and cooking techniques), juicing, detoxification, and supplements. This is your new way of eating and living—every day, all week, all year long. The new you. No more eating cheap, fake, junky crap. From now on, you're eating real.

Later in this book, we'll go beyond food and talk about mindfulness, managing stress, and the importance of physical movement. We'll also discuss how to be a savvy patient, build your Whole Health Team, and take full command of your health.

Eating Real

Eating real is all about *ease and simplicity*.

You don't need to measure exactly four ounces of oats. You don't need to be fussy and obsessive about portions and calories. You don't need to spend twenty hours in the kitchen, bent over a hot stove, following complicated recipes with dozens of ingredients. We're going to keep things simple, quick, fresh, and tasty.

What to Eat

For the rest of your life, I want you to eat:

+ Real food, which means organic vegetables and fruits, and whole, unrefined grains and legumes. Aim for abundance and diversity—at least thirty different types of produce every week.

You can do it! Use this handy checklist to help you increase the diversity of foods you eat.

1. Apples
2. Artichokes
3. Asparagus
4. Beetroot
5. Bok Choy
6. Broccoli
7. Brussel sprouts
8. Cabbage—red and green
9. Carrots
10. Cauliflower
11. Celery
12. Celery root or Celeriac
13. Chard
14. Chicory
15. Collard greens
16. Corn
17. Dandelion greens
18. Dates—soaked
19. Eggplant
20. Endive
21. Fennel
22. Garlic
23. Grapefruit
24. Grapes
25. Green beans
26. Kale—all varieties, cooked only
27. Leek
28. Lettuce—all varieties except Iceberg
29. Melons
30. Onions
31. Oranges
32. Parsley
33. Parsnip
34. Peas
35. Peppers—green, red, and yellow
36. Potatoes—all varieties
37. Pumpkin
38. Radish
39. Shallot
40. Spinach—cooked only
41. Squash—all varieties
42. Sweet potato
43. Tomatoes
44. Turnip
45. Watercress
46. Yams
47. Zucchini

✦ Juices made from organic fruits and vegetables.

What NOT to Eat

✦ Food that has a label on it.

✦ Food that was prepared in a factory.

✦ Food that has been contaminated with toxins/pesticides.

+ Food that has been heavily processed—frozen, freeze-dried, deep-fried, preserved, sulfured, packaged, etc.

+ Food that has been sitting on a shelf for more than two days, like packaged crackers, cookies, breads and cereals.

+ Food that is refined, like flours, oils, beverages, etc.

+ Food that feels hard to digest, or that just doesn't feel "right" for your body. Anything that leaves you feeling sluggish instead of energized. (Everyone's body is slightly different, so pay attention to how you feel after each meal to see what's working for you and what's not.)

+ Foods that you are allergic or sensitive to. Give your body one week on this program and then you can try to reintroduce those foods. Several of my clients overcome their allergies quickly. Of course, if your allergies are anaphylactic, please don't try to reintroduce the foods those foods on this program. Consult a doctor or allergy specialist before taking any serious risks.

+ Foods that are coated in refined salt, sugar, or oil.

+ Foods that have a face or a mother (hint: fish, seafood, or meat).

"Whoa! But Where Will I Get My Protein?"

That's the first question everyone asks me when they learn about this program. I'll summarize the answer quickly below, and I invite you to read *Proteinaholic* by Garth Davis, MD, if you are really concerned about getting enough protein.

1. You've been misled for decades, by the meat, dairy, and agricultural industry, about the amount of protein your body needs to maintain health.

111

2. More is not better. In fact, too much protein, like the volume consumed in our SAD (Standard American Diet), actually shortens your life span.

3. You don't actually eat "protein." You eat essential amino acids found in food, which your body then uses to build thousands of different types of proteins that your body requires. This process happens inside your body.

4. The largest land animals on the planet are herbivores and eat only plants: the giraffe, elephant, buffalo, bison, cattle, moose, horse, rhinoceros, hippopotamus, and even a number of extinct dinosaurs, too.

5. You can be a high-endurance or even an ultra-endurance athlete, like Rich Roll and others, and still live an entirely plant-strong lifestyle.

6. Animal protein is low in fiber and quality minerals and vitamins and high in calories, fat, pesticides, hormones, and antibiotics.

7. Certain proteins found in milk have been linked to the onset of many chronic diseases, including cancer.

8. It's almost impossible to become protein-deficient, unless of course you are trying to starve yourself and eating too few calories per day, or you have a rare genetic disorder, digestive imbalance, or inadequate stomach acid that prevents you from digesting proteins adequately. If you are eating a variety of whole plant-based foods, you'll find you are getting all the protein you need.

Digest this information above and lettuce dive deeper into the food details later in this book. Yes, all puns are intended.

Use Common Sense

You don't need to be a scientist, a health expert, or an orthomolecular nutrition educator to know what "real food" is and isn't. You already know.

A fast-food cheeseburger? Not real food.

A fruit-flavored energy drink that's full of mysterious chemicals? Not real food.

A salad topped with stale croutons, cheese crumbles, and strips of processed deli meat? OK, we're moving in the right direction, but that's still not real food.

Real food is clean, unprocessed, wholesome, and close to nature—the kind of food that you can pluck from the garden or pick off a tree.

A good question to consider is, "If I eat [insert food here], will this promote health, or will this take away from my health?" Use your common sense to guide you.

Stop Counting Calories

Yes. You'll never need to count another calorie again. And you'll also get to eat when you are hungry and as much as you want. That's because the Gerson Therapy, many plant-based lifestyles, and this program in particular are based on eating a plethora of whole foods that are naturally high in nutrients and low in calories. The standard American diet is full of processed and refined ingredients and is typically low in nutrients and high in calories, which forces you to consume even more food, as your body and brain are desperate to get quality nutrients that will support their many daily functions.

And don't worry, you won't go hungry with this new lifestyle. In fact, you'll find that your energy is sustained for longer periods of time between meals—no more energy dips at 11:00 a.m. and 2:00 p.m., and no more food cravings at night.

Though I don't like to market the *Eat Real to Heal* program as a weight-loss plan—if I did, I'd be a billionaire—I will warn you that the weight will melt off of you, even with you exercising less and eating more!

Bye-bye yo-yo diets, gimmicky packaged weight-loss programs, and infomercial exercise gadgets purchased late at night.

Hello crazy sexy healthy new body that you feel and look amazing in—and all you need is a juicer, a kitchen knife, an enema kit, and a great relationship with a local organic farmer.

Eating Real: A Sample Meal Plan

Here's what a day of real food could look like...

Breakfast: A beautiful bowl of cooked organic, rolled oats. Cook it slowly, over low heat, adding plenty of water so it's not dry. Add fresh or stewed fruit.

Lunch and dinner: A baked potato, a cup of Hippocrates Soup (recipe on page 83), and a beautiful leafy green salad with an abundance of chopped or shredded vegetables or fruits and homemade salad dressing. Slow-cooked veggies, like onions, tomatoes, butternut squash, and collard greens, that you'll cook using the "long and low" method (meaning, cooked for a long time over low heat), and a delicious baked dish of beets, cauliflower, and turnips, and you are good to go.

Juices: Sip organic fruit/vegetable juice throughout the day. If you're adhering to a strict Gerson Therapy protocol because you have a life-threatening chronic disease, the Gerson prescription is thirteen-eight-ounce juices-a day—

basically, one glass every hour. That's the recommended amount for serious diseases like cancer, because we want you to keep pumping nutrients into your body and flushing toxins out of your cells and tissues. However, if you're not battling a life-threatening disease like cancer, heart disease, or other illness, then the five-week *Eat Real to Heal* program invites you to try consuming three—eight-ounce juices—a day.

Dessert: Peach crumble with a touch of cinnamon and nutmeg, or creamy, frosty, homemade banana nice cream.

Those are just a few ideas, of course. Feel free to add your own creative flair!

Later in this section, you'll find cooking techniques and lots of real food recipes, too.

Eat Real 2 Heal Meal-Breakfast

Prep tips + How to plan your food?

A. Herbal tea, eg. Peppermint or chamomile

B. Orange or grapefruit juice (for breakfast only) green juice carrot juice carrot/apple juice

C. Use thick rolled or steel cut oats

D. Prepare 1 to 2 types of fruit & stew for 20 min while cooking oats, keep on low temp with lid on, no water

Eat Real 2 Heal Meal-Lunch & Dinner

Prep tips + How to plan your food?

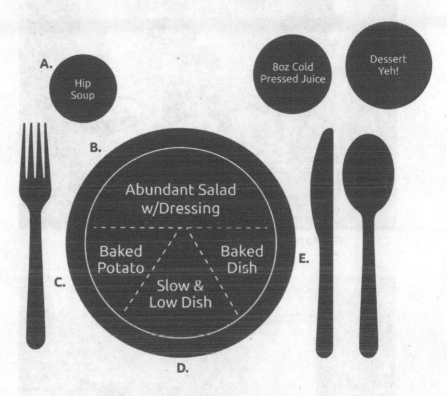

A. Hip Soup

B. Abundant Salad w/Dressing

C. Baked Potato

D. Slow & Low Dish

E. Baked Dish

8oz Cold Pressed Juice

Dessert Yeh!

A. Follow instructions for Hippocrates Soup

B. Prepare a variety of raw greens & finely chopped, raw veggies enjoy w/salad dressing

C. Red, yellow, russet, gold, etc. Bake on low temp mashed is okay w/chopped herbs, onions, garlic, ACV, flax oil or dressing

D. Prepare tomatoes, onions and 1 to 3 other veggies, layer in pot with airtigtht lid, no water & cook slowly on low temp for 1 hr

E. Prepare 1 to 4 veggies, and bake on low temp

Getting ready to serve a delicious healing meal at our
wellness center in Pemberton, BC.

Gathered with our Nutrition and Detox Train the Trainer Students. About to
enjoy a plant-strong meal made with love.

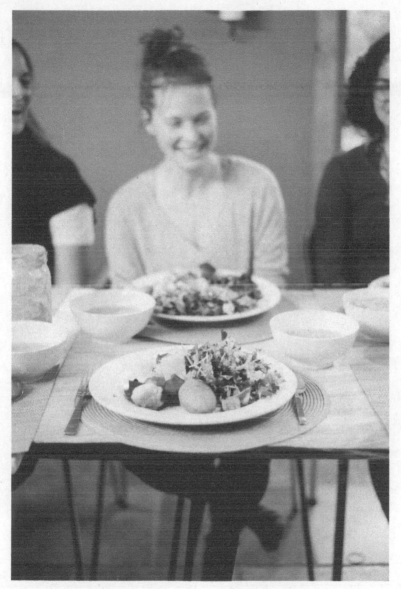

Both food and laughter are truly the best medicines.

"Those who eat together stay together." —Author unknown

The Power of Eating Real

Even Bones Heal Fast

A while back, one of my daughters had an accident and injured her arm. We rushed her to the emergency room to be examined.

Her doctor assessed the situation. She had broken the head completely off her radius bone, and she definitely needed surgery followed by a cast. My daughter sat there calmly throughout the X-ray and the examination. She wasn't comfortable, but she wasn't in agony, either.

The doctor pulled me aside to chat, and said, "It's incredible that your daughter is so calm. With this type of injury, most people experience lots of swelling, and they're in excruciating pain, causing them to scream in pain. But your daughter doesn't seem to be in very much pain."

A few weeks later, that same doctor remarked that the healing process had moved along beautifully. Almost a year faster than expected! "Everything's looking perfect," said the doctor.

A few weeks after that, my daughter was totally back to normal, playing and running outside, and doing cartwheels, and the X-ray showed no lingering trace of the injury or even the break.

The doctor seemed surprised by my daughter's rapid healing process. But I wasn't surprised—because this is the power of eating real, clean, nutrient-dense food.

When you're fueling yourself with real food, pain and inflammation are decreased, even non-existent. Injuries heal faster. All of your body's systems function in top form. Your body can be the healing machine that it's designed to be.

My daughter, May 29, 2017, two hours after breaking her arm.

Hazelle's X-ray during surgery, May 31, 2017.

Hazelle and me feeling good post-surgery, June 1, 2017.

Hazelle swimming cast-free, no pain, fully healed, July 3, 2017.

Cooking Techniques

Long and Low

For optimum health, you want to cook your veggies using the "long and low" method. This means cooking slowly, for a long time, at a low temperature and with no added water. So, rather than cranking up the heat and scorching your veggies, or steaming or boiling the nutrients out of them, you're going niiiiiiice and slow.

Why do this? It's all about getting the most nutritional bang for your buck. When you go long and low, you're using heat to break down parts of vegetables that would otherwise be indigestible, and you use heat to make the phytochemicals more readily available so that your body can absorb the maximum amount of nutrients from every bite.

By cooking without water in the Long and Low method, you keep many of the valuable water-soluble vitamins from migrating into the boiling water, which means more nutrients available to you.

One of my favorite long and low dishes is a simple pan of tomatoes, onions, garlic, butternut squash, and collard greens.

+ Wash all of your produce.

+ Peel the skin of the squash and scoop out the seeds.

+ Peel the onion.

+ Leave the skins on your tomatoes.

+ Remove the chunky stem of the collard greens.

+ Chop everything into large chunks.

+ Toss everything into a stock pot.

✦ Put an airtight lid on the pot.

✦ Cook on medium heat until the pot is hot to the touch or filled with steam, or the veggies start "sweating," and then turn down the heat to the lowest setting.

✦ Cook over low heat for sixty minutes—or longer, if necessary.

✦ If your stove runs extra-hot, place a heat diffuser between the pot and the element to drop the temperature a further few degrees.

✦ If you find you don't quite have the technique right at the beginning and your veggies are burning, then you can add a small splash of water if the veggies are sticking to the sides of the pan. But try to get the technique of sweating your veggies to produce the moisture your dish needs to not cause a burning or sticky mess.

✦ Keep the air-tight lid on your pot at all times so as to not let the steam escape.

✦ After sixty minutes, you'll have a beautiful pan of soft, stewed veggies that are positively jam-packed with nutrients and flavors that your body will love.

✦ Top with a delicious dressing or eat as is.

When you're done cooking your veggies, you might notice some extra liquid in the pan. This is liquid medicine—don't throw it away! You can drink it straight from the pan, add it to a pot of soup, shake it into a salad dressing, or add it to your next glass of juice.

Water Frying

Did you know that you can "fry" veggies without using butter or oil? It's true.

It's all about using the long and low method. You can practice with an onion. Peel off the outer layer of brown, papery skin. Chop it up. Toss it into a saucepan. Cook it long and low. Stir occasionally. If your onion begins to stick to the sides of the pan, add a few tablespoons of water. Not too much. Just a tiny bit. Keep stirring. When the onions start sticking again, add a few more tablespoons of water. Keep stirring. Eventually, you'll have a beautiful pan of deep, rich, buttery, caramelized onions that look and taste like they've been fried, even though you haven't added a single drop of refined oil.

Baking

As a busy parent who also runs five different businesses, baking is a life-saver! I love baking veggies because you can chuck things into the oven, set a timer, and walk away. You don't have to hover over the pan. You can go do something else and let the oven work its magic.

Here's how I do it. I gather together a bunch of veggies— squash, onions, potatoes, carrots, whatever I've got—and gently wash everything in filtered water. Always leave the edible skins on the fruits and veggies and be careful to not scape away the skin while washing them, as many of the valuable nutrients live just below the skin's surface. Then I chop the veggies into chunks. They don't have to be perfectly uniform. Imperfection is fine! I toss everything onto an oven-safe glass or stainless-steel dish, plop it into my preheated oven (around 275–350° F or 177° C), and bake for about sixty minutes. Every oven is different, so get to know your oven intimately. Use the lowest temperature that will allow you to bake veggies until tender within sixty to ninety minutes.

Firm veggies (like potatoes) need to bake for the full sixty minutes. Softer produce (like zucchini and squash) take less time, more like thirty minutes, depending on how thickly you've sliced them. I never worry about timing my dishes perfectly. I simply toss everything in and enjoy them as they turn out.

Once I can poke the veggies with a fork, they're done. Just like that, I have a huge pan of veggies that I can use in a variety of ways—tossed into a salad, pureed into soup, rolled into a lettuce wrap, or in a bowl with a dressing or sauce. So many possibilities!

Soups

I follow these steps when making the kidney-cleansing Hippocrates Soup, or any other soup recipe.

+ Wash the ingredients

+ Chop veggies into large chunks—they'll either be blended or milled, or will break down into smaller sizes while cooking, so don't waste your time cutting them into bite-size pieces

+ Place all ingredients into a large soup pot

+ Fill the pot with distilled or filtered water to the same height as the top of the veggies. This will always give you a wonderful soup consistency. If you like your soups thicker, or more like a broth, then add less or more water

+ Mill, blend, or eat soup as is

Note: Always use the food mill and mill the Hippocrates Soup, and NEVER blend it, as blending will distort its delicious flavors. Other soups, like a savory squash-leek soup, could be blended or eaten chunky.

My Favorite Recipes

These are a few real food recipes that I make every week, They're tried-and-true favorites in my household. I hope they become go-to favorites in your home, too!

SNAZZY BAKED POTATO

This is one of my favorite lunches—quick, easy, and tasty. I usually bake a dozen potatoes at a time—right on the oven's wire rack, no baking tray needed—and keep them in the fridge so my family can grab them quickly.

Ingredients

1 potato; cooled
A few teaspoons of flaxseed oil (NEVER EVER heat or cook with flaxseed oil—always consume it at room temperature or colder)
A few teaspoons of apple cider vinegar
A handful of chopped veggies and herbs (celery, bell pepper, basil, anything you want)

Directions

Wash and gently scrub a large potato. Poke the skin with a fork a few times. Bake until it's fork-tender—usually about sixty to ninety minutes at 350° F (177° C).

Split open the potato, let it cool off slightly, and drizzle a bit of flax oil and apple cider vinegar on top. Add your favorite veggies—I love to use chopped celery, chopped red bell pepper, chopped onion, minced garlic, and fresh herbs.

All done! It's like a zingy salad tucked inside a potato.

DR. G'S BASIC DRESSING

This is delicious drizzled on a green salad, baked potato, baked vegetables, pretty much anything. Your taste buds will rejoice—and your body will, too.

Apple cider vinegar is full of potassium, magnesium, and probiotics that help your body function optimally. If you struggle with digestive issues—including acid reflux— definitely give this dressing a try.

Ingredients

⅔ cup freshly squeezed orange juice (approximately five oranges)
¼ cup apple cider vinegar
½ cup flax oil
2 T maple syrup
½ bunch parsley
¼ medium-sized red onion

Directions

Juice the oranges and add the juice to the jar. Wash and chop the parsley. Finely dice the red onion. Toss all of that into the jar, too. Add the apple cider vinegar, flax oil, and maple syrup. Screw a lid onto the jar and shake until nicely blended. Or whirl everything together in a blender, if you prefer.

For a variation, try replacing parsley with a few chives. Add some grated ginger for a zippier recipe. Or, substitute grapefruit juice for orange juice, or try a mix of several citrus juices.

YAM NINJA DRESSING

This can be used as a salad dressing, a dip, a sauce, anything you want. For starters, try tossing this dressing into a bowl of grated or shredded cabbage, carrot, apple, and jicama to make a delicious, crunchy slaw. Delicious— and so nutritious, too.

Yams are rich sources of Vitamin C, which helps your body fight infections, heal from injuries faster, and has many other benefits.

Ingredients

1 medium-sized yam (roasted) (about one cup)
⅓ cup freshly squeezed orange and lemon juice (two oranges, one lemon)
⅓ cup apple cider vinegar
⅓ cup flax oil
¼ cup water
2 cloves garlic
1 inch ginger
2 green onions

Directions

Scrub the yam to remove dirt. Bake in the oven until tender—usually about forty-five to sixty minutes at 350° F (177° C). Peel and discard the skin. Cut into chunks. Meanwhile, juice the oranges and lemon. Peel the garlic and ginger. Slice and reserve the green onions. Put all of the ingredients—except the green onion—into your blender. Blend until smooth. Add sliced green onion at the end.

AND THE BEET GOES ON...

This is a vibrant salad dressing with an intense pink color—thanks to the beets! Drizzle this dressing over your favorite veggies, and get your phone ready, because you'll definitely want to snap a photo for Instagram.

And let's take a moment to celebrate the wonder of beets! Beets are packed with Vitamin C, potassium, manganese, and folate. These humble roots carry so many benefits for your body—healthier nerve and muscle function, stronger bones, and a happier liver, kidneys, and pancreas, not to mention decreasing the risk of birth defects. They simply can't be beet!

Ingredients

1 large (or 2 small) beets
1 large apple
⅓ cup freshly squeezed lemon juice (2 to 3 lemons)
⅓ cup apple cider vinegar
½ cup flax oil
2 T maple syrup

Directions

Preheat the oven to 350° F (177° C). Wash the apple and beets and slice them into quarters, making sure to discard the apple seeds and stem. Add some liquid to the bottom of a roasting pan or casserole dish. Roast the apple and beets until soft—approximately 30 minutes. Juice the lemons. Add all of your ingredients to a blender—including the liquid from the roasted apple and beets. Blend until creamy and smooth. If you like, you can add some fresh chives at the end.

SIMPLE LETTUCE CUPS

Here's a crunchy, tasty salad that looks lovely, too. If you've got a few extra apples lying around, this is a great recipe to use them up. This recipe serves one, but feel free to double, triple, or quadruple the ingredients to make a bigger batch. Serve this to your dinner guests, and they will be impressed!

Ingredients

1 green apple
1 carrot
A few teaspoons of apple cider vinegar
A few teaspoons of flax oil
Butter lettuce leaves

Directions

Using a grater or a mandoline slicer, shred your apple and carrot into ribbons. Toss with vinegar and oil. Add fresh herbs if you like. Spoon the mixture into a butter lettuce leaf—they're nice and round, almost like a cup or a small bowl. Voilà! Salad cups!

HIPPOCRATES SOUP

Hippocrates was a Greek physician who lived from 460—370 BC. He was one of the first physicians who believed that diseases are caused by environmental factors, including eating and lifestyle habits—not caused by angry, vengeful gods, as many ancient Greeks believed. He is considered to be one of the fathers of modern medicine.

Hippocrates Soup was Dr. Max Gerson's favorite soup for disease prevention and recovery. It's a staple in my household, and it couldn't be easier to make. You can double the quantities in this recipe if you want to make a big, family-sized batch or keep some extra stock in your fridge to use as a base for yummy sauces.

Ingredients

4 stalks of celery
1 parsley root (if you can't find this at your grocery story, no worries, you can skip it)
½–1 pound of tomatoes
2 onions
2 leeks (or substitute with 2 more onions)
1 pound of potatoes
A handful of fresh parsley
A couple cloves of garlic

Directions

Remove the skin from your onions. Wash and scrub your veggies. Chop coarsely. Simmer in a big pot—long and low heat, very slowly—for about two hours. You can eat the soup just as it is, or you can puree it with a food mill. Store in the refrigerator and enjoy within two days.

RED PESTO

This recipe comes from Jennifer Just, a Green Moustache team member and nutritionist. (Jennifer recently became the very first Green Mo' franchisee, and she runs the Green Mo' cafe in Squamish, British Columbia. She's a rock star.)

Jennifer used to struggle with anxiety around public speaking, like so many of us do. Once, in the middle of a cooking class, her hands started trembling uncontrollably. She was demonstrating this exact recipe—Red Pesto—and she was worried that everyone in the room could see her wobbling and trembling.

The class ended and Jennifer thought, "Yikes. Well, that was a complete disaster." But, actually, it wasn't! The students were totally impressed with this recipe and gave Jennifer a huge thumbs-up, and lots of praise, and told her they loved the class.

Moral of the story? Sometimes, all you need is a tasty recipe to turn a disaster into a triumph! Jennifer loves using this Red Pesto sauce on baked potatoes or spooned on top of veggies.

Ingredients

6 small beets
¼ cup flax oil
3 tablespoons lemon juice
1 medium cooked potato
2 cloves of garlic
A handful of fresh basil

Directions

Wash, scrub, and chop the beets into chunks. Cook the beets slowly—long and low, in a covered pot—with a small amount of water until they're nice and soft. It will take 30-40 minutes, depending on how big your chunks are. Let the beets cool. Toss them into your food processor or blender with the remaining ingredients. Pulse until smooth.

CABBAGE SLAW WITH ORANGE DILL VINAIGRETTE

A member of the Brassica family, this leafy vegetable comes in many varieties. Green, red, savoy, and white are the most commonly found in the grocery store. This beautiful vegetable is full of Vitamins C, K, and B6, manganese, fiber, and potassium.

Cabbage slaw is easy and quick and can be either a side or a main dish. It is inexpensive and delicious to eat at any time of the year. Here is a simple recipe that you can prepare in large quantities and enjoy the leftovers the next day or on those days when you feel a little pressed for time.

Ingredients

¼ head red cabbage, shredded
¼ head green cabbage, shredded
1 or 2 celery stalk(s), sliced
½ red onion, thinly sliced
3 radishes, thinly sliced
¼ cup orange juice
2 tbsp apple cider vinegar
¼ cup flax oil
1 tbsp. chopped dill

Directions

In a mixing bowl, combine all the vegetables.

Whisk the orange juice, apple cider vinegar, flax oil, and dill together and drizzle over the cabbage slaw as much as you desire.

You can sprinkle some fresh herbs on top for extra flavor.

Chill in the fridge for an hour to allow the flavors to meld together and enjoy!

"ANYTHING GOES" HUMMUS

Hummus is traditionally made with chickpeas, but anything goes! Instead of chickpeas, you can use baked potatoes, baked beets, baked squash, just about anything that will add some thickness. This is a great dip, sauce, and spread that pairs beautifully with pretty much any veggie.

Ingredients

A baked potato or other baked veggie of your choice
Some chopped garlic
A splash of flax oil
A splash of lemon juice

Directions

For this recipe, don't worry about measuring everything precisely. Just wing it!

Grab your blender and drizzle some flax oil into it. Add some chopped garlic and lemon juice. Then, add your baked potato (or baked beets, baked squash, baked parsnip or lentils that have been cooked long and low). Blend until thick and creamy, like a spreadable paste. Add a touch more oil if necessary, or a bit of water.

APPLE CRUMBLE

A delicious breakfast, snack, or dessert. You can remove the apples and swap in some peaches, plums, or any fruit you want.

Ingredients

1 handful of organic oats
1 apple
A few pinches of cinnamon and nutmeg
Dash of honey, maple syrup or molasses

Directions

Cook the oats in some water, long and low, to soften them slightly. Slice your apple or cut into chunks. Layer the oats and apple in a small baking pan. Drizzle with maple syrup. Sprinkle your cinnamon and nutmeg on top. Bake at 350° F (177° C) for ten minutes or so, until the apples have softened up.

BANANA NICE CREAM

Directions

If you've never had vegan banana (n)ice cream, prepare to have your mind blown. It's so easy to make, you don't even need a recipe. Just peel a few bananas, chop into small pieces, and freeze them (this is the only time you can freeze your food in this program). Then toss the frozen chunks into your blender—ideally, a super-strong blender like the Vitamix or Blendtec. Whirl until frosty and smooth. It will form a thick cream that tastes like vanilla ice cream.

Please note that I'm not a chef. For me, food is medicine. Food is also fuel. Most importantly, food must be healthy if it's to be consumed at all. Because I choose to make my life exciting outside of the kitchen, I tend to spend as little time in the kitchen as I have to. However, I know that some of you readers LOVE being in the kitchen every moment of the day. So, here's where I recommend purchasing the *Gerson Cookbook*, as it was developed by a Gerson Chef and is the most comprehensive and accurate cooking guide in the history of the Gerson Therapy. It's like having a Gerson Chef in your kitchen!

It has step-by-step instructions, over 150 mouth-watering recipes with colorful pictures and helpful tips, and more.

. . .

Hundreds of Additional Recipes

For hundreds of additional plant-strong whole-food recipes to REVERSE cancer and chronic disease, check out...

✦ *The Gerson Therapy Cookbook*[4]

---

4 Available for purchase on the Gerson Institute website: https://gerson.org/gerpress/

+ *The Gerson Institute Website*

+ The Green Moustache blog[5]

+ The Green Moustache Salad Dressing Cookbook (coming soon)

There are hundreds of anti-cancer and chronic-disease cookbooks that I could recommend, but I don't want to overwhelm or confuse you. Several other anti-chronic-disease books still recommend a high intake of sodium salt, protein, and hard-to-digest foods like nuts, seeds, meat, and avocados, and refined sugars and oils. The *Eat Real to Heal* book, combined with Charlotte Gerson's book *Healing the Gerson Way* and the Gerson Therapy cookbook will provide you with all the information you need. Plus, it's the cleanest, realest way to get healthy fast.

Time-Saving Tips

Short on time? Can't labor over a hot stove for hours on end? Got other things to do?

I can definitely relate! With five businesses, three kids, and two very active dogs, efficiency is essential in my kitchen.

My personal strategy is to block out a section of time—say, one and a half hours every two days in the evening—and, in that time, I do all the cooking/meal prep for all six meals, for all five family members, for the next two days. It's perfect. I actually spend less time in the kitchen preparing six meals than if I tried to prepare them one or two meals at a time.

There's actually a lot that you can accomplish in one and a half hours. For starters, you can roast an entire pan of potatoes, two baked dishes, and an apple crumble in one

---

5 https://www.greenmoustache.com/juicyblog/

go. Use the potatoes in a variety of ways—bowls, salads, sauces, and so on.

While everything is baking happily in the oven, you can do something else—like, wash and chop up the Hippocrates Soup and get that cooking.

Next, you'll want to get your Long and Low-cooked dish stewing on the stovetop.

After that, you can whip up two or three salad dressings, store them in glass Mason jars, and chuck them into the fridge, so that you're all set for the days ahead.

Lastly, you could wash and prep a bunch of apples, carrots, and all of the ingredients for your green juice, arrange everything in reusable containers, and stick it all into the fridge, so you have ready-to-go ingredients to make juices that evening and the next day. Note: Don't cut up your juicing ingredients in advance—simply wash and group them into portioned recipes, so that all you have to do is pull them out of the fridge, cut them up into smaller juicer-size pieces, and then juice away.

You could do all of that...and you'll probably still be finished before your baked dishes are finished!

ou choose simple recipes with less than ten ingredients and minimal steps—like the recipes featured in this book—cooking becomes much speedier and easier. You'll be amazed by how much you can create—and how little time it takes!

But I Already Eat Really Healthy!

Once, a client—let's call her "Rebecca"—came to see me with a chronic health condition.

"I eat super-healthy all the time," Rebecca told me. "But I'm constantly tired. I just don't feel good, and I can't figure out why."

We had a chat about her eating habits, I took a full health history from birth to her present age, and she described what a typical breakfast, lunch, and dinner would be. Right away, I could see the issue. Rebecca was eating lots of "healthy" cereal and granola, "healthy" protein bars, "healthy" frozen burritos, "healthy" canned soups, "healthy" oatmeal cookies, "healthy" hummus and sauces, and so forth.

Yes, she was sticking to organic food, which is great. But her meals were mostly comprised of pre-packaged foods— stuff from a box, from a can, from a plastic container, stuff produced in factories, stuff loaded with too much salt, sugar and refined oils. Rebecca wasn't eating many fresh fruits and veggies. She thought she was eating "super healthy," but in fact, her body was nutrient-deficient—that's why her energy levels were slumping.

I encouraged her to switch to real food. "Ditch the processed stuff for five weeks," I advised her. "Eat real food, straight from the garden. Let's load your body with organic fruits and veggies and some grains, though in much smaller quantities than what you are used to. I bet your energy levels will totally change."

She did. And it worked.

I've had hundreds of clients and customers just like Rebecca over the years. People who feel "pretty good, but not great." People who aren't exactly "sick," but aren't thriving and vibrant either. If that's your situation,

I encourage you to look closely—and honestly—at what you're eating. You might feel like you're sticking to a super-nutritious diet, but...maybe not! Switch to real food and—just like Rebecca—you'll feel a big difference.

But What about Protein?

Yes, we are going to tackle the protein conversation one more time, just so I know that you and I are speaking the same language before you begin this five-week *Eat Real to Heal* challenge. In the list of recipes that I just suggested, you might have noticed that none of them include meat, eggs, avocado, dairy, nuts, or seeds, or any other forms of animal or rich plant protein.

This is because we don't need as much protein as we've been led to believe. In fact, too much protein is very tough on the body. Oh yes, the beef industry has worked hard to convince you that meat is crucial for strength and vitality! But it's simply not true.

If you look online, you'll see several blogs written by vegan weightlifters, vegan boxers, vegan bodybuilders, dancers, Iron Man athletes, and marathoners who are all living—and thriving—without meat. They stick to a plant-based way of eating, and they're functioning in top form, because of their plant-strong lifestyle. If they can, why not you?

Just as an experiment, stop eating animal protein for five weeks. Notice how you feel. Taking a "meat break" is a beautiful gift for your kidneys and your cells. You'll allow them to circulate excess sodium effectively through your body while flushing out excess water and acidity, which can build up over time from too much protein. After eliminating animal or high-protein foods for five weeks, you might feel lighter, more energized, and have a clearer head. You might not miss pork chops as much as you thought you would. As I say to my clients, "Nothing tastes as good as healthy feels."

If you're curious to learn more about the science of protein—and how we've been duped into thinking we need to eat tons and tons of it to be "healthy"—check out a book called *Proteinaholic*[6] by Garth Davis, MD.

But What about Salt?

A lot of clients ask me, "Can I sprinkle some good-quality salt onto my meals?" You can—but I'd strongly recommend that you don't. Why? Because most of us consume way too much salt already.

Health organizations recommend no more than 2,300 milligrams (about one teaspoon) of salt per day. But most people in North American consume far more than the recommended amount—and the consequences are severe. Excessive salt intake spikes your blood pressure, which, over time, increases your risk of having a heart attack or stroke. Yikes. Kind of makes you think twice before sprinkling extra salt on your veggies, right?

If things "just don't taste right" without extra salt, that's because you've grown accustomed to a high-sodium diet, and your taste buds need a little time to adjust.

If you reduce your salt intake for a short time—even just ten days—then you'll give your taste buds a chance to adjust, and your palate will change. After two weeks or so, you'll notice that you don't "need" the excess salt anymore. Things will taste amazing without it!

And What about Alcohol?

You've probably seen the headlines that say, "Red wine contains antioxidants that can fight cancer!" and "Moderate alcohol consumption is good for your heart!" and so forth.

6 http://proteinaholic.com/

Is it true? The jury's still out. Some studies say yes, and others are inconclusive. Dealing with alcohol is one of those situations where you need to view your body as a living laboratory and pay close attention to how things impact you.

When you have one glass of wine, how do you feel the next morning? What about two glasses? What about none?

Rather than buying into the media hype—or trusting the latest news headlines—trust the information you're receiving from your own body. Ultimately, that's the information that matters most.

Whether you choose to consume alcohol or not, I definitely recommend moderation, and I recommend taking a break every now and then—especially if you're recovering from an injury or battling a disease. You want to remove everything from your body that puts extra stress on it. And give your hardworking liver a break, rather than giving your liver even more work to do.

When you drink alcohol, similar to when you consume too much protein, salt, sugar, or oil, your body puts all other systems on hold in order to use its energy to eliminate the excess alcohol, salt, protein, sugar and oil before any of it can damage your organs and tissues. Often, this process of elimination and self-regulation to maintain homeostasis can take four to six hours. And then, around 12:00, lunch begins, and your body is back to cleaning up the mess once again. This means that your body never gets the break it needs to focus on healing, repair, and regeneration, which leaves it in a tired, even exhausted state. When you eat the foods described in this book, you'll simply allow your body to consume the highest amount of clean, organic nutrients with the lowest impact on your being, leaving you feeling energized, light, and vibrant.

If it feels really difficult to stop drinking alcohol for five weeks—or even for five days—you are not alone. There are millions of people who don't necessarily fit the description of "alcoholic," but who feel somewhat dependent on alcohol, and who'd like to cut back and find other ways to unwind and de-stress. Check out Hip Sobriety for inspiration and like-minded people. You can also hire a therapist or counselor, join AA, or find help within your church group or another spiritual center. If you want to cut back on alcohol, or abstain completely, there are millions of people who are on the same path. Join them. You don't have to walk alone.

Healing Reactions

When you quit eating processed food, you're giving your body a tremendous gift. After about five weeks, you will see and feel all kinds of positive changes. But at first, especially during that very first week or two, things might feel...a little weird.

Some of my clients—not all, but some—experience what I call "healing reactions." Other people call these "detox symptoms." These are unpleasant—but very temporary—reactions that you experience while your body is detoxifying, healing, and adjusting to your new way of eating.

Detox symptoms can include feeling inflamed, feeling bloated and gassy, headaches, wicked bowel movements, or feeling soreness in your joints, especially in places where you've had an injury or surgery previously, including breast implants or metal plates on your bones.

Why? What's happening is that your body is going into "healing overdrive." Now that it's being flooded with nutrients, your body thinks, "Hooray! Now we can really get to work and do some serious healing and repair." Your body starts working extra-hard to repair damaged cells, tissues, and organs, which can cause inflammation and soreness. But again, it's only temporary.

With a healing reaction, typically, it hits you like a ton of bricks, but by twenty-four to seventy-two hours later, it's totally gone. It's not like a cold or flu that creeps up slowly. A healing reaction is more like a quick flare-up and then, whoosh, it's all gone.

Don't be worried if you feel some healing reactions. It's a good thing—and it's a sign that your body is healing. That said, always trust your instincts. If you're feeling "off" and your instincts say, "Something is definitely not right," then plan a visit to your doctor ASAP.

Doing coffee enemas, which help manage pain and inflammation and assist the liver in detoxifying the body, is necessary to lessen or eliminate the healing reaction flare-ups.

We discuss coffee enemas in greater detail on page 115.

A Few Tips for Parents

You're excited to eat real. But your kids...maybe not so much?

Maybe your kids are accustomed to ordering from Pizza Hut for dinner. Maybe they're hooked on mac 'n' cheese from a box—the kind with that nuclear orange powdered cheese. Maybe they're used to getting donuts from Tim Hortons as a reward for doing well at school. Or maybe your kids are willing to eat fresh fruits and veggies, but only certain types—bananas are cool, maybe blueberries, but everything else? Forget it.

As a parent, you're the primary role model in your kid's life. It's up to you to lead by example, and to show your kids that eating real food can be fun, tasty, and satisfying.

Visit our Sea to Sky Thrivers website—the non-profit arm of our businesses—Richer Health blogs, or sign up for one of my workshops for more ideas on raising healthy kids.

As well, here are some pointers that might help:

1. **Don't try to trick your kids.**

   I've seen parents try to trick their kids into eating veggies by hiding cauliflower florets under a pile of mashed potatoes, for example. It's not going to work. Your kids are too smart to fall for tricks and gimmicks!

   Trickery is not the solution. A better option is to get your kids involved in shopping, washing, chopping, and making meals at home. The more you involve your kids in the process, the more interested and enthusiastic they will be.

   You can also help your kids to grow a garden. Plant some herbs on the window sill. Bring the kids to the market and let your toddler pick out her favorite yellow, orange, and red heirloom tomatoes, whichever ones she likes best. Get them involved, and they'll be way more likely to eat what you're serving.

2. **Remove the competition.**

   You can't have competing foods in the house. If there's a bag of salt and vinegar chips in my house, my kids will always choose those over the healthier, more satisfying options. All those cheese strings, Cheerios, Goldfish crackers, and sleeves of Oreos— they have to go, or your healthy-kids wishes will never come true.

   This doesn't mean you can't have any fun snacks or treats. You can! Just upgrade to high-quality, nutritious treats.

For example, you can make date bars by mixing soaked dates, rolled oats, and cinnamon in a food processor and then shaping them into small bars. Sweet and quick! Or try my super-simple three-ingredient banana oatmeal cookies—banana, oats, and cinnamon mashed together and baked until tender. Try a banana shake made with oat milk. During hot summer days, puree, in a blender, fresh fruits like mango, peaches, or watermelon mixed with a bit of orange juice, and place into ice pop molds to give you a tasty refreshing treat. It can be that simple, and it's fun to re-discover the real, simple taste of a freshly cut sliced apple, banana, or peach. You can also stew fruits and blend them into sauces. Applesauce is still my fourteen-year-old daughter's favorite dessert to make—one ingredient...blended stewed apples. Delicious!

Bottom line: if you dump the junk and replace it with real food, you and your kids will both have an easier transition into this new lifestyle. Set yourself up for success!

3. **Don't pressure, bribe, or bully your kids into eating their veggies and fruits.**

It's just not necessary to do this. Most kids won't starve themselves. Eventually, they're going to get hungry, wander into the kitchen, and ask for something to eat.

If eating real food is a totally foreign concept, they might grumble a bit at first. They might throw a little tantrum. But if you serve real food consistently, day after day, pretty soon, they'll get on board. They'll see you chopping fresh, crunchy veggies. They'll inhale the aromas of simmering squash, garlic, and onions. They'll hear the whirring sound of the juicer and blender, and they'll watch beets and carrots being transformed into colorful pesto, sauces, and soups. Soon, all of this will feel normal and natural.

Just think of the tremendous gifts that you're giving to your children: The gift of top-quality nutrition. The gift of healthy habits, from a young age, so that they don't have to make a challenging transition when they're older. The gift of strength and health. They're worth it. So are you.

Mindful Eating

Food is medicine. Food is fuel. However, food is also so much more than that.

Food can be a community celebration—a chance to gather and make memories, a time to talk about what happened in your day, to connect deeply with loved ones, or if you're eating alone, to connect with yourself. Mealtime can be a rushed, frenzied experience, or it can be done in a very mindful way.

I grew up in a household where mealtime was pretty rushed. We always ate nourishing, homemade food. However, once the food was on the table, it was total mayhem! My three younger brothers and I would dive in, grabbing spoonfuls of curry, rice, and veggies as rapidly as possible. The situation was, basically, how fast can you get to the food before somebody else takes it away?

Needless to say, this type of rapid-fire eating is not ideal. It's emotionally stressful and it's tough on our digestive systems, too. I've had to learn, as I've gotten older, to slow way, way down at mealtime. One bite. Pause. Another bite. Chew thoroughly. Another bite. Smile and say a little internal blessing ("Thank you, food") for your meal. Pause. Chat, laugh, and share stories. Then another bite. When we eat slowly and mindfully, it changes the entire experience. Food tastes better, for starters. And also, you'll improve the digestive process, which means you'll absorb even more nutrients from every bite.

Food is one of the greatest pleasures in life, and it's a pleasure we get to enjoy three to six times every day. The keyword is "enjoy." What would make mealtime feel more enjoyable for you? What would help you to slow down and really savor the experience? Maybe lighting a candle. Playing soft music. Or using the "nice, fancy china" instead of saving it for "someday later." Why can't "someday" be today?

For the rest of today, I encourage you to eat your food extremely slowly and mindfully—so slowly that it almost feels silly. At first, it will feel weird. You'll probably feel like a cow in a field, chewing in slow motion. Some people might wonder what's wrong with you. Don't worry about them, though! Focus on enjoying your food. Eating mindfully is also about being aware of "just eating," experiencing flavors, textures, and temperatures, and being aware of the thoughts in your head while eating.

Then, consider how you can slow down and be mindful in other aspects of your life, too. Perhaps you can be a little more mindful in how you take a shower, fold laundry, make your bed, drive to and from work, and ride your bike. Slow down and feel the wind on your skin. Slow down and appreciate the morning sunlight pouring through your bedroom windows. Slow down and notice the extra two inches of height that your daughter suddenly has—she's growing up so strong, so fast! Slow down long enough to say "thank you" to a hardworking colleague or beloved friend. Slow down to feel more joy.

Most of the times, we're rushing-rushing-rushing around like maniacs, and our brains are swirling with a million different thoughts. Practicing mindfulness simply means that you're bringing your mind into the present moment— slowing down and focusing on one thing, not a hundred things. This is the most enjoyable way to eat—and live. Try it, and feel the difference.

From Miscarriage To Miracle

Years ago, a woman hired me for nutrition counseling. She's a client I will never forget.

All she wanted was to have a child. She'd been trying to get pregnant for a long time, and it had been an intense struggle. Finally, just when she thought her dreams would come true, she experienced yet another miscarriage and lost the baby. Her doctor comforted her but couldn't provide any answers. "These things just happen," she was told.

My client's doctor told her that she was healthy, and she could try for another pregnancy. But my client wasn't so sure. She was also forty-three years old. She suspected that something was "off," and she pushed for more testing. It turned out, she had uterine fibroids. These are non-cancerous, benign tumors that grow in the uterus. They are not life-threatening, but they can cause pain, pressure, cramping, and other issues. To get rid of them, doctors typically recommend medication, embolization (which involves using a catheter to inject tiny particles into the fibroids to destroy them), or hysterectomy, in which the uterus is completely removed and getting pregnant is completely out of the question.

My client wanted to try a different approach. She came to me, seeking a non-surgical treatment option for the fibroids, and maybe, possibly, a path to having a child. I explained that upgrading your diet can be tremendously helpful—it's not a guaranteed fix, but it can definitely help. She agreed to try.

I helped her get on a real food plan, following the Gerson Therapy recommendations. Thirty different fruits and veggies every week. Fresh juice several times a day. Detoxifying techniques, including daily coffee enemas.

Supplements to nourish her body even more. Clean, filtered water. Rest. Gentle movement and exercise.

After six weeks, her fibroids had shrunk down to 50 percent of their original size. After twelve weeks, they were gone completely. Another four weeks after that, she was pregnant. Today, her child is five years old. Some might call this a "miracle." I call it the power of real food.

I have hundreds of client success cases like the one above—not just for infertility and fibroids, but for hundreds of different types of chronic illnesses and cancers. *Eat Real to Heal* is a specific program for a host of non-specific chronic illnesses caused by two things—nutrient deficiency and toxicity. Reverse those two factors, and you reverse your disease.

I know people who've spent $30,000 to $100,000 in their quest to feel better, to reduce pain, lose weight, get pregnant, or beat disease. Thousands of dollars on prescription medications, surgical procedures, infertility treatments, weight-loss regimes, and more. And yet, the greatest gift you can give to your body costs almost nothing at all. All you need is a basket of organic produce, an open mind, and the willingness to fuel your body with real food.

Food is one of the most powerful forms of medicine we have, and it's also the most overlooked and forgotten. It's time to reclaim the healing medicine that's already inside your fridge, garden, or local grocery store. Before you resign yourself to a child-free life, before you give up on beating diabetes, before you decide that feeling mediocre is "as good as it's going to get," make a significant change to your eating habits. Eat real. Watch what happens next. It could be downright miraculous.

All about Juicing

We've spent a lot of time talking about cooked food, and now we're getting into...

Juice, juice, wonderful juice!

Drinking fresh, organic vegetable and fruit juice is one of the most efficient ways to saturate your body with nutrients.

You don't want to sit down and eat ten to twenty pounds of vegetables. That would take forever, and you'd feel stuffed and bloated afterwards! But with a juicer, you can take ten to twenty pounds of produce and distill everything into eight-ounce single portions, consumed several times throughout the day. So much plant-power streamlined into a single beverage. It's truly liquid gold.

How Much Juice?

Personally, I aim to have one to three glasses of juice every day. Each glass should hold about eight ounces. When I have a client who's battling cancer and doing the Gerson Therapy program, their protocol will be bumped up to thirteen glasses a day, one every hour.

What Goes Into It?

Nature's bounty! You can make juices from a variety of ingredients. In the *Eat Real to Heal* Program, you'll consume one to three glasses a day of the following staple juices.

1. The Green Juice, which is made up of leafy greens such as romaine lettuce, tart apples like Granny Smith apples, green peppers, purple cabbage, inner beet greens, chard, endive, and watercress.

> Note: DO NOT use kale, collards, or spinach in your juice—these greens are better consumed cooked and with their fiber intact.

2.   The Carrot-Apple Juice, which consists of just that, carrots and apples.

For breakfast, you can also include one hand-squeezed eight-ounce citrus juice of your choice: orange, grapefruit, or a combination of both.

After you have completed the five-week *Eat Real to Heal* program or the Gerson Therapy, and only after you are fully healed, you can begin to get creative with your juices and juice ingredients. As you can see, your juices can be really simple—just one to two ingredients—or wildly abundant—six ingredients or more.

For the *Eat Real to Heal* program, and when doing the Gerson Therapy, stick to the specially formulated juice recipes to maximize healing.

When Is the Best Time to Drink the Juices?

Spread them out throughout the day. You can sip one glass at each meal—breakfast, lunch, and dinner. If that doesn't work for you, you might have a green juice in the morning, followed two hours later by a carrot juice, followed six hours later by a carrot-apple juice.

Whatever schedule you want to do is fine—as long as you're spreading them out throughout the day. Don't chug them back to back. Spreading them out allows your body to take in all the water-soluble nutrients, while not being too flooded by all those nutrients. If you drink them all at once, you end up excreting lots of water-soluble vitamins and losing the benefit of the juices.

Store-Bought or Homemade?

You can purchase bottles of cold-pressed, organic juice from a store or juice bar. But at $8 to $12 per beverage, that can get very pricey. If you're drinking one to three glasses a day, it adds up! That's why I recommend investing in a juicer and making your own juice at home. Plus, it's guaranteed fresh—it's always best to drink your juice within fifteen minutes of making it. Most juice bars don't have the luxury of offering you this service. If they did, you'd be waiting hours for a juice.

What about Doing a Juice Fast?

A "juice fast" or "juice cleanse" or "juice detox" is where you stop eating solid food and only drink juice, typically one to seven days in a row.

I don't recommend doing this. It's very trendy right now—and some people swear that they feel amazing doing it—but I've found that it does more harm than good for those suffering from a chronic health condition.

The problem with a juice fast is that you're not getting fiber, healthy fats, essential amino acids, necessary carbohydrates, or any of the other building blocks that your body needs. It's beneficial to consume those every day, and they all help with eliminating toxins. Juice fasting may be beneficial for a short period of time for someone who is not suffering from a chronic disease and who is also being carefully monitored by a health professional skilled in the science of fasting. My recommendation is: keep on juicing, but eat actual food, too!

My Favorite Juicers

I love the Norwalk. It's the king, or queen, of all the juicers. It's about $3,300 CAD ($2,959 USD) to purchase the machine. It's a serious investment, but, just like a car, this is a machine that you will use every single day, and it will last a lifetime. And unlike many other juicers, it's super-easy to clean.

If you feel like, "That's a ludicrous amount of money to spend on a juicer! No way!"...well, I get it. But here's the funny thing. Most of my clients usually start off with a lower-end juicer. They'll purchase one for, say, $149.

Then, after a few weeks, it gets jammed. Or they get sick of cleaning it because it's fussy and difficult to take apart. So then they purchase a stainless-steel juicer that costs a little bit more money, but the juice is foamy and they're not getting enough liquid into each glass. Then they purchase a third juicer, or maybe even a fourth. By the end of it, they've spent the exact same amount of money as if they'd just gone ahead and purchased the queen of juicers: the Norwalk (named after Dr. Norman Walker, 1886–1985, who healed himself and lived to be ninety-nine years old using juicing, quality nutrition, and food as medicine).

I'm not saying, "You must go out there and buy the Norwalk." You do have other options.

A few juicers I love are the Hurom, the Omega, the Champion, the Green Star, and my favorite next to the Norwalk, the Angel, which is also stainless steel but costs far less than the Norwalk. The Angel is a masticating twin-gear juicer, which means that it has two shafts that look like screws that sit next to each other. Your produce goes through while the shafts spin, and it crunches up your vegetables and presses out the juice through a fine stainless-steel mesh component. It's a fantastic juicer that runs about $1,000 to $1,200 CAD.

Whatever juicer you choose, take good care of it. Treat it like a piece of medical equipment. Clean it thoroughly after each use. Keep the warranty packet in case you ever need to get it repaired. Replace the smaller bits if they get worn out. With care, your juicer will work hard for you, and last a long time.

If you still feel uncertain about making this kind of investment, remember the cost per use. If you go for, say, the Angel, you'll be spending about $1000. If you make two glasses of juice every day, that's 730 glasses per year, which means the cost per use is just $1.36 per glass, plus the produce to be juiced for that first year. And your Angel will last for many, many years. Now, compare that to the price of a meal at a fancy restaurant, or a nice outfit that you may or may not ever wear again, plus all the other "one-time-use" or maybe even useless things we purchase in any given year to make ourselves feel good for fifteen minutes, but that have no effect on preventing, managing, let alone reversing, a chronic illness.

Stainless Steel versus Plastic

What I like about stainless-steel juicers is that you can take them apart, rinse them in water, and put them on the shelf to dry. Very easy clean up.

Plastic juicers? Not so great. Some of the plastic juicers can get cracked over time. The minerals from your juice can stick to the plastic, and you have to scrub it vigorously to be able to get it clean. They also tend to get jammed and stuck more than the steel ones. I'm not saying the plastic juicers are totally useless—some are pretty decent—but personally, I'd go for steel.

Go for Quality

Like I mentioned earlier, it's tempting to purchase the cheapest juicer on the market—but this can lead to clogged pipes, annoying clean-up situations, frustration, and then spending more money later down the line, regardless!

I advise you to purchase the highest-quality juicer that you can afford right now. Go for the high end, not the low end. Just like purchasing a great mattress for your bed—where you'll spend eight hours a day, every day—a great juicer is one of those investments that will upgrade your quality of life every day.

Preparing Your Produce for Juicing

Before juicing, you want to wash your produce thoroughly.

Grab your vegetables and wash them well in a clean sink

full of filtered or distilled water. Please, no vegetable cleaning sprays or chemical-laden cleaning products. Just soak them in water for a couple minutes, or rinse under running water. No need to scrub. You don't want to scrub away the skin of your veggies or apples because there are plenty of valuable nutrients just under the skin.

I like washing my veggies in filtered water, because chlorinated tap water is full of chlorine and other harmful organic and inorganic materials. What's the point of making a beautiful glass of juice if it's contaminated, right?

After washing, chop your produce into chunks, and remove the cores from your apples so that it will all pass through your juicer more easily. Some of the top-notch juicers are super-strong, and you can throw an entire carrot inside and it will juice it up, no problem, and no chopping required. But for the budget juicers, you'll want to chop things up to prevent jamming the machine.

Using Your Juicer

No matter what kind of juicer you're using, be gentle! You don't want to shove or force the vegetables down. This will cause annoying jams and breakdowns and will also cause your juice to foam.

Let the juicer slowly take in the produce. Of course, always make sure you have a cup, glass, or bowl under the spout so all the juice gets collected. If your juicer produces a lot of foam, just skim it off.

Drink your juice right away, ideally within fifteen minutes. The fresher the juice, the more nutrition you'll get.

Drinking Your Juice

Just like mindful eating, it's best to practice mindful juicing and sipping. Don't chug your juice to get it down as fast as possible. Slow down. Enjoy your juice. Let it swish around in your mouth, really taste it, before swallowing it. This will activate your salivary glands and your digestive system. Sip slowly so that all the nutrients can get absorbed into your body effectively. Cheers!

Nutrient Absorption

There is a saying: *You are what you eat.* However, that's not exactly true. You are what you *absorb*.

One of the main reasons people get sick is that they're eating plenty of food, but they're not absorbing nutrients well. This can be because the food hasn't been cooked enough (it's totally raw and hard to digest) or the opposite—it's been heavily processed in a factory and the nutrients have been sapped out. It can also be because your body has been weakened over time and you lack the digestive enzymes and acids to break down your food into easy-to-absorb rations.

This is why I encourage my clients to consume a mixture of juice plus food that's been cooked long and low. In terms of nutrient absorption, these are your best options. The supplements that we'll discuss will also help you better digest and absorb invaluable nutrients from your foods and juices.

Juicing removes all of the fiber from fruits and veggies while leaving the nutrients intact. When we drink juice, nutrients travel through the body through osmosis, get absorbed into the system quickly, and are utilized by the mitochondria in all the cells, tissues, bones, and all parts of the body. Lots of nutrient absorption, very little waste.

And then there's the long and low cooking method, which we talked about before.

With the long and low cooking method, we use heat to break down the fibers in the food for maximum nutrient absorption. The food is almost "pre-digested" with the heat.

When we eat this food, it is almost like eating baby food. The food is cooked for a long period of time. Some people refer to it as mushy. I tend to refer to it as stewed— decadently stewed, so that it melts in your mouth with every single bite.

Detoxification

Meet the Mighty Liver

Lift up your right hand. Place it on the right side of your body, halfway up from your pelvis and below your chest. That's where your liver lives.

Your liver is a mighty organ that does so many phenomenal things. It's responsible for over five hundred functions. It keeps our body clean, healthy, balanced, and detoxified. When your liver is overwhelmed and not functioning correctly, you've got big problems.

Many people don't realize that the liver is partly responsible for balancing hormones. When we think about hormone balancing, we might think about the thyroid, the hypothalamus, and the pituitary gland in the brain. But the liver is also responsible for balancing hormones. For starters, it produces a hormone called sex hormone binding globulin, or SHBG, which is a protein that is responsible for trapping excess hormones in our body, dissolving them, and essentially spitting them out of the body so we have the right balance of estrogen—which keeps other hormone levels, like progesterone and testosterone, in balance. And two out of three breast cancers are hormone-receptor-positive, meaning that they grow in response to estrogen.

If your liver is sluggish and not working well, then it can't produce enough SHBG to keep your estrogen levels in check. This means your estrogen levels will increase and affect the levels of other hormones. For this reason, and many others, it's imperative to keep the liver happy, detoxifying, and healthy.

Give Your Liver Some Love

Many years ago, I enrolled in a yoga teacher training program, which included a section on human anatomy.

When we began learning about the liver, our instructor stood up, placed her hands on her liver, and said:

"Repeat after me: Hello, liver. Today I will take every action to keep you healthy and clean, and allow you to do what you're meant to be doing without bogging you down."

She encouraged us to stand and recite these words right there in the classroom, and do so every morning.

This may seem a bit silly—talking to your own liver, seriously?—but it's a beautiful thing to do. You can do it first thing in the morning, or right before bed. You can lie down. Close your eyes. And then say aloud, or privately, inside your mind, "Thank you, liver. Thank you for taking good care of me. I promise to take good care of you, too."

Powering Up Your Liver

If you've been eating a typical North American diet for most of your life—lots of processed food, lots of salt, lots of preservatives, lots of non-organic fruits and veggies— then your liver is, quite frankly, over burdened. And your microbiome isn't doing well, either. It's been overloaded for too long. Picture an office worker with a thousand unread emails and twenty urgent project deadlines who's been working nonstop for decades. That poor employee is probably one email away from a nervous breakdown. That's how your liver might be feeling right now.

To power up your liver, you want to switch to real organic food and drink your juices—things we've already discussed in this book. These lifestyle changes will help to flush out your system and give your liver a much-needed break. Before too long, your liver will be humming along nicely, and able to do its important work without being overloaded.

To power up your liver even more, I recommend doing a coffee enema once a day for five weeks in a row. To further support your liver, take the nutritional supplements.

Introducing: The Coffee Enema

I know what you're thinking.

Coffee? Enema? As in, I'm supposed to put coffee up my butt? Excuse me, Nicolette, but have you lost your mind?!

I know it might sound pretty wacky, but please bear with me. It may sound peculiar, but this is one of the most efficient ways to cleanse your liver, ridding your body of toxins that have built up over the course of many years, even decades.

How It Works

A coffee enema is not the same as a colonic. With a colonic, you are shooting large amounts of water inside of you to scrub your insides clean. That's not how a coffee enema works.

With a coffee enema, you are targeting your liver, up through the hepatic portal vein. The coffee hits the liver and, thanks to the caffeine and palmitates in the coffee, stimulates it to create more bile and trap toxins. Then, those trapped toxins run through your digestive tract and out through your colon and rectum.

The History of the Coffee Enema

Early in his career, Dr. Max Gerson was treating a few patients who had cancer. Sadly, these patients died. During autopsies, Dr. Gerson discovered that the cause of death

was hepatic coma. This is the hardening of the liver.
It happens when the liver becomes so burdened and
sluggish that it solidifies and becomes hard like a rock.
The liver is overloaded with flushed toxins and it becomes
ineffective. The liver cannot perform any of its functions
anymore. This leads to death.

In these autopsies, Gerson was surprised to discover that
he couldn't detect the cancer. The immune system had
been able to attack the cancerous tumors successfully—but
meanwhile, the liver was failing. In a sense, these patients
died from liver failure, not from cancer.

Max Gerson wondered, "If I could have found a way to
reactivate the liver and get it working again, perhaps these
patients would have lived." He began experimenting with
different strategies to power up the liver, including coffee
enemas, and had great success.

How to Perform a Coffee Enema

Ingredients

An enema bag or bucket

A large stainless steel cooking pot

Organic ground coffee (light roast is best, because it
has the highest caffeine levels)

A metal tea strainer to catch the coffee grounds

An old towel

Filtered or distilled water

Directions

1. Put four cups of water in a pot and bring it to a
gentle rolling boil.

2. Add three heaping tablespoons of coarsely
ground coffee.

164

3. Let it boil with the lid off for three minutes.

4. Place the lid on the pot and turn the heat to low.

5. Let the coffee mixture gently simmer for 12 minutes.

6. Pour the mixture through a metal tea strainer into a glass Mason jar.

7. Let the mixture cool down to a comfortable temperature. Warm, but not too hot. Think body temperature or a baby's milk bottle.

8. Set up your bathroom while the mixture cools.

9. Lay an old towel or blanket on the floor, on top of a yoga mat or Thermarest, in your bathroom.

10. Clean your enema bucket and hose. Once cleaned, close off the clamp on the hose.

11. Pour the body-temperature coffee mixture into the bucket (aren't you glad you closed off the hose clamp?).

12. Place a non-toxic lubricant around the first five inches of the tube's tip.

13. Open the clamp and let the air inside the tube escape so that coffee fills the tube, then close the clamp again.

14. Lie down on the towel on your RIGHT side.

15. Insert the end of the tube roughly four to five inches inside your rectum.

16. Place the bucket of solution 18 inches above your waist.

17. Open the clamp and the solution will drain in. If it does not flow, try deep breathing, raising the

bucket higher, twisting the inserted part of the tube slightly, or moving the tube out and then back in a few millimeters.

Releasing the Enema

18. Hold the solution for 12 minutes, or until you feel a strong urge to release the enema. Eventually, once all the toxins are released, you'll find it easier to hold for the entire 12 minutes, though there is no reward for holding it shorter or longer periods of time. Use this time to read a book, meditate, do visioning exercises, or simply rest...

19. After 12 minutes, release the enema solution into the toilet, clean up with a gentle soap or cleanser, and hang the bucket so that the tube and the hose dry thoroughly.

Further Hints

+ If you develop a cramp, close the clamp, turn from side to side, massage your belly, place a hot-water bottle on your belly, hum, or take a few deep breaths. A cramp usually passes quickly.

+ If possible, do the enema after a bowel movement to make it easier to retain the coffee. If this is not possible, take a plain water or chamomile enema first, if needed to clean out the colon.

+ If intestinal gas is a problem, some exercises before the enema may eliminate the gas. Deep belly breathing will also help.

+ If water will not flow around the entire colon, try gently massaging your lower abdomen.

+ If the enema makes you jittery, reduce the amount of coffee or solution for one week, then try again with the full-strength solution.

✦ Eat something before doing a coffee enema to activate bowel movement. Eat something small after taking the enema too.

✦ Ensure the enema is at body temperature for comfort. Always check whether the water is too hot or too cold. You can even use a cooking thermometer to get really precise.

✦ Be patient, as practice makes perfect.

✦ Stay warm and cozy. Keep yourself comfortable and warm by using a blanket and pillow.

How Often?

I recommend doing a coffee enema once a day for five weeks in a row. If you want to seriously commit, you can even do it twice a day—morning and night—for five weeks. Think of this like hitting a reset button for your liver, and by extension your entire body.

Note: The ratio of juices to coffee enemas is this:

Drink three eight-ounce glasses of juice for every coffee enema you do in a twenty-four-hour period. Therefore, if you drink six eight-ounce glasses of juice, you would do two coffee enemas in a twenty-four-hour period, and so on.

You're activating your liver, powering it up, getting it back into top form. It's like taking an athlete who's been out of shape, stiff, tired, in retirement for many years and...boom! We're getting that athlete ready for a comeback tour!

After five weeks, you may consider doing fewer coffee enemas. BUTT—yes, the pun was intended—I highly recommend you keep this wonderful detox activity included in your life. You will feel the typical toxin burden feelings when you need an enema: foggy brain, aching joints, tired, etc. Some of my clients will do a weekly coffee enema for maintenance. Others do it once a month. It's up to you. However, please note that, every day, your body is taking in and eliminating waste and toxins. Supporting your liver with daily or weekly coffee enemas is simply good hygiene. You do brush your teeth daily, don't you? Why not do the same for your mighty liver?

A Few Other Detoxification Techniques

Coffee enemas are fantastic! I can't sing their praises highly enough! I love teaching people how to do enemas at home, because I've seen how effective they are, and I've seen the life-changing (sometimes, life-saving) benefits of detoxifying in this way. Yes, I'm a proud enema advocate. I should get a t-shirt that says "Ask Me about Enemas," although I'm sure that would horrify my teenage daughters.

However, enemas aren't the only detoxification technique. There are many others that you can try in addition to the wonderful coffee enema. Here are a few that are really easy to do, and you probably have the necessary materials in your kitchen already...

Tongue Scraping

Have you ever woken up, looked in the bathroom mirror, and seen that your tongue is coated with a slimy white film? All that gunky stuff is toxic residue—dead cells, sometimes stinky bacteria that causes bad breath, plaque buildup, and other stuff—that's trying to escape your body. Don't swallow it! You want to scrape it off and get it out.

Tongue scraping is an Ayurvedic practice that's been done in India for many centuries—and recently, it's becoming more popular in Western countries too.

To do it, simply take a small metal spoon, flip it over, reach into your mouth, touch down on the back of your tongue (as far as you can go without gagging), and gently scrape towards the tip of your tongue. You can also purchase a special U-shaped tongue scraping tool on Amazon (get a copper one, not a plastic one), but most people find that a plain old spoon works just fine.

Tongue scraping is a good way to remove unwanted bacteria, wake up your taste buds and encourage them to regenerate, and also stimulate your salivary glands, which leads to effective digestion.

Who knew you could do so many positive things for your body, all with a humble spoon?

Oil Pulling

Do NOT do this if you have cancer. Much like tongue scraping, Oil pulling is really simple to do. I like to do it first thing in the morning right after I wake up, just after or before I scrape my tongue.

Simply take one tablespoon of organic, unrefined, cold-pressed coconut or sesame oil. Put the oil into your mouth. Don't swallow it, but swirl it around in your mouth for ten to twenty minutes. You can stroll around, make your bed, boil water to make your oatmeal, do some juicing, or stretch, as you're swishing the oil around, pushing and pulling it through your teeth and along your gums.

Let the oil get warm and melty. Get it up into your gums, around the roof of your mouth, everywhere. Swish, swish, swish. Think about pulling the oil back and forth across— and through—your teeth. The oil is pulling bad bacteria out of your mouth.

After ten or twenty minutes, you will feel a frothy mixture in your mouth. Spit it out into an organic waste bin, as it will tend to clog up your sink, and then brush your teeth. This might be strange at first—some people don't like the fatty, oily sensation—but you will get used to it, and it's incredibly good for your body. It eliminates bad breath better than any mint, mouthwash, or other product on the market. Afterward, your mouth will feel sparkling clean!

Try doing this once a week. Some people even do this daily, but once a week is definitely better than never.

Lymph Massage

Another way to detoxify is by doing lymph massage. You don't need to hire a massage therapist to do this—you can do it yourself!

Before your morning shower, take your right hand, place it on your left shoulder, then slide it down your arm briskly, like you're waking up your arms. Repeat a few times. Repeat on the opposite side. Then repeat on both of your legs, underneath your ribs, underneath your breasts or chest, up your throat and the back of your neck.

By brushing and pulling on your skin, you're activating the lymphatic system, a network of tissues and organs that purge toxins out of your body. One of the main functions of the lymph system is to transport infection-fighting white blood cells around your body. So, if you've got a sluggish lymph system, that means it's harder for the white blood cells to travel around and fight disease. You don't want a sluggish, sleepy lymph system. You want it wide-awake and activated.

That's why lymph massage—sometimes called lymph drainage—is a great daily practice. You can do it with your bare hands, or you can use a loofah or body brush, or wear exfoliating gloves or mitts, to add a little extra friction. Google "exfoliating shower gloves" and choose a non-toxic brand that's made from bamboo rather than plastic. You can pick up a pair for $5 and use them over and over.

In addition to massaging yourself, you can also try tapping. My mother-in-law is a massage therapist. I learned this technique from her. To do it, you stand up and start gently tapping all the way from your face down to your arms, up your arms, underneath your armpits (your beautiful lymph glands are located there), on your chest, down your legs, all the way down to your toes. My kids love it when I do this to them, and they'll do it to me. It really wakes you up and gets the circulation moving.

Clay Packs

If you suffer from joint pain, or any kind of painful inflammation, you're going to love using a clay pack.

What is a clay pack, you ask? It's another simple, inexpensive detoxifying technique that you can whip together at home.

First, you need some fabric—an old, soft, clean flannel shirt is great. Cut your fabric so you have a big square or rectangle. Then you need some therapeutic clay. Google "Bentonite Clay"or "Montmorillonite clay."You can purchase a big one-pound jar from the Gerson.org website and from other online retailers.

In your kitchen or bathroom, mix the clay powder with filtered water, following the instructions on the back of the jar. Pour the liquid clay mixture into your fabric. Allow it to absorb all the way in. Now you have a clay pack.

You can place your clay pack onto a sore joint—say, your knee—and wrap it around your knee, letting the clay-soaked fabric press directly onto your skin. Let it rest there for as long as you can. An hour or two is great, but if you're pressed for time, take a shorter resting period. Read a book, watch an inspiring movie, or chat on the phone with a friend while your clay dries.

It's a bit messy, so you might want to do this outside, or while lying on a towel. I like to place the clay-soaked fabric on my skin, then layer a dry piece of fabric over that, and place and then wrap it in plastic wrap. That helps to contain the mess a bit.

Why do a clay pack? Clay packs are powerful because they do double duty—clay magnetizes toxins and draws them out through your skin, and it also deposits minerals into your body, like calcium, magnesium, iron, potassium, silica, copper, chromium, and zinc.

Have you ever met a pregnant woman who felt a strange craving to eat clay or dirt? This was something I encountered in all three of my pregnancies—I really wanted to eat dirt! Why? Most likely because I was craving minerals and nutrients that I couldn't get enough of through my diet. Clay contains a lot of those essential nutrients we need. So, try a clay pack instead of munching dirt from your garden.

Castor Oil Packs

A castor oil pack is basically identical to a clay pack, except you're saturating your fabric with castor oil instead of liquid clay.

Warm up some castor oil, pour it all over your fabric, drench it, get it really soaked in.

You can place the pack on your back, on your stomach, over your liver (if you don't have liver tumors), on your kidneys, anywhere that feels inflamed and painful. If you suffer from PMS bloating and/or cramps, place a castor pack on your lower belly. Many of my clients experience total relief after doing a castor pack for an hour. You can lie down and fall asleep with it on. The longer you leave it on, the better.

Castor oil is edible, too. Depending on your age, you might remember your grandparents—or even your parents— telling you "Take your castor oil!" whenever a flu bug was going around. It doesn't taste great, that's for sure, but it's powerful stuff.

Between coffee enemas, tongue scraping, oil pulling, lymph massage, clay packs, and castor packs, you've got a serous detoxification arsenal. Your body will say "thank you" a thousand times over, especially your hardworking liver.

Now that we've discussed how to pull toxins from your body, next, we're going to talk about how to replenish your body with minerals and vitamins that you need.

Yes, you'll get most of these nutrients from your food and juices, but even if you maintain a super-amazing diet, there might be a few gaps that we need to fill in with natural, organic supplements.

Supplements

Imagine a room with one hundred people in it.

Most likely, here in North America, ninety to ninety-five of those people have some type of nutrient deficiency.

Often, you can fix a nutrient deficiency by simply upgrading your eating habits. Switch from snacking on Cheetos to eating collard greens, carrots, and quinoa, and boom! Problem solved. But sometimes, you need a little extra help because your body is in a very weakened state and food alone isn't enough. Also, some nutrients are difficult to get from food alone. That's where taking supplements can make a big difference.

Which Supplements? How Many?

Which supplements should you be taking, if any? This is a tough call, because everyone's body and medical history is unique.

You'll need to work with your Whole Health Team—your physician, your nutritionist, your naturopath and other health providers, and of course, yourself—to track your symptoms and figure out if you have any deficiencies. Most likely, you do. It's just a matter of figuring out which ones.

If you're eating real food, drinking juices every day, detoxifying your body regularly, and getting enough rest, and you still feel tired, sluggish, or just "not right," then that's a sign that you probably have some type of deficiency.

Which Kinds of Supplements?

You want supplements with no fillers, dyes, flavorings, or artificial ingredients. Just a plain capsule filed with the nutrient you need. That's it.

You can get big jars of supplements from a compounding pharmacy. These will be much, much cheaper than buying them from Whole Foods or a health-food store. You can also order them online. A few websites that I recommend can be found on the Gerson.org website, under Supplements.

What's Missing?

These are some of the most common nutrient deficiencies in North America and other Western countries:

Acidol Pepsin

Acidol pepsin helps to increase the level of hydrochloric acid (HCl) in your stomach. HCl is needed to break down food in order to absorb nutrients. If you don't have enough HCl, it makes it really hard to digest food.

That's why when somebody comes up to me and complains about digestive issues (bloating, constipation, feeling sluggish), one of the first things I typically recommend is taking some form of acidol pepsin supplement. It works wonders!

B12

B12 is important for mitochondrial function, cellular metabolism, and many other processes in our bodies. Unfortunately, if you're eating a plant-based, meat-free diet, then you're probably not absorbing enough B12 from your food. Grab a supplement—they are cheap, effective, and absolutely necessary for plant-based eaters, and even meat eaters, as most of our foods today are too clean, meaning all the good bacteria as well as the bad bacteria have been stripped away.

Note: Always use methylcobalamin, never cyanocobalamin.

CoQ10

CoQ10 is an enzyme that's needed to keep our metabolism and heart working properly. Much like B12, it's mainly found in animal products like meat—especially heart, liver, and kidney organs. So, if you're sticking to a plant-based, meat-free diet, then you'll probably want to add a CoQ10 supplement into your routine.

It's often recommended to take your CoQ10 supplement along with a spoonful of flax oil. One researcher, Karl Folkers, found that when you dissolve CoQ10 in flax oil before swallowing it, you'll absorb the enzyme much more effectively. Cancer patients should minimize oil intake.

Iodine

We need iodine in every single cell of our body. One of iodine's functions is to trigger apoptosis, which is programmed cell death. When apoptosis isn't happening, our cells don't die on cue, and that's a terrible thing, especially if our normal cells become mutated. We also need iodine to keep our thyroid, liver and skin healthy.

Some of the symptoms of iodine deficiency are depression, headaches, fatigue, memory issues, and menstrual problems. You can eat lots of iodine-rich foods—seaweed and other sea vegetables, cranberries, strawberries, potatoes—but that is generally not enough to reverse the deficiency, as most foods are not grown in iodine-rich soils anymore. Lugol's solution is my favorite household iodine supplement brand.

Niacin (Vitamin B3)

Dr. Abram Hoffer was a researcher who studied people who were institutionalized and diagnosed with schizophrenia. He found that many of these people were depleted in key nutrients, especially niacin. When he supplemented these nutrients in very high doses, he was able to fully reverse the symptoms of schizophrenia. These patients could return back to society. (He wrote several books about his studies, and they're amazing. Definitely worth checking out.)

Niacin and Vitamin B3 are the same thing. When you take niacin, usually within thirty to sixty minutes, you will feel your whole body getting warm, flushed, tingly, and possibly even itchy. This is normal. It's called "the niacin flush," and it's a good thing, not a bad thing.

What's happening is that the B3 is dilating your capillaries, allowing more blood to flow through, which means more oxygen and nutrients are being carried around your body. The flush is temporary, not dangerous, and it will pass pretty quickly.

Potassium

Potassium is a mineral that works with sodium to keep your electrolyte levels in balance, regulate your heartbeat, and prevent muscles from cramping. Potassium and sodium are a power duo, like Bonnie and Clyde, or Beyonce and Jay-Z. The problem is, most people consume way too much sodium and way too little potassium. We need to bring things back into balance.

If you've got a potassium deficiency, you might notice symptoms like tiredness, cramps in your larger muscles (especially your arms and legs), and nausea. You can get potassium from foods like apricots, artichokes, bananas, and beans. But if that's not enough, try some supplements, too.

Supplement, Not Substitute

It's important to remember that supplements are not a substitute for real food.

I know it might sound crazy, but I've met plenty of people who think, "Oh, I can eat burgers and poutine and drink tons of beer, and it's OK. I'll just take my supplements to make sure I'm getting all the vitamins and minerals that I need."

Nope. That's not how it works. You want to fuel your body with top-quality, organic, plant-based food and juices first, and then, if necessary, you can add supplements into your regime. But it's exactly that—a supplement, not a substitute.

Use Your Body as a Living Laboratory

You don't need to rush out and buy all of the supplements that I just mentioned. You might not need all of them.

Again, I recommend starting with the basics that we've already discussed: Switch to real food, sip juice once to three times a day, detox using coffee enemas, get plenty of rest, and manage your stress levels as best you can.

Do that for five weeks in a row. Then evaluate how you feel. Think of your body as a living laboratory. You're a scientist in the lab, assessing all kinds of factors—your energy levels, your pain levels, your inflammation/puffiness/bloating, your PMS symptoms, your sex drive, and so on.

After five weeks, if you're still feeling fatigued, or if you're grappling with frustrating symptoms that don't seem to be improving, then it might be time to start exploring the world of supplements.

Measuring Your Progress

One of the most exciting things about upgrading your eating and lifestyle habits is that you can see and feel positive changes almost immediately.

I always encourage my clients to measure their progress closely so they can really see what's happening in their bodies. When you see, for example, that your cholesterol levels have dropped significantly, and your blood sugar is back in balance, all in just five or six weeks, WOW! That's thrilling information, and it is proof that this is really working!

After seeing that kind of proof, most people feel even more enthusiastic and committed. They tell me, "OK, now I get it. This is really helping. I can see the results. I want to stick with this new lifestyle...for life."

There are lots of different ways you can measure your progress. Here are a few recommendations:

+ Ask your doctor to do a blood test (cholesterol, blood sugar, red and white blood cell count, thyroid levels, all of your hormones) before you start making any kind of food or lifestyle changes. Get a baseline assessment of where you are right now. Then repeat the same blood test five weeks later, after you've diligently followed the guidelines in the book for all of those weeks. Compare the results. Most likely, you and your doctor will see a big difference.

+ Check how your clothes fit. Take before and after progress pictures. If you're trying to lose excess fat, water, and bloating, switching to real food will help you do that. If you're trying to build strength and muscle, switching to real food will help you do that, too.

+ If you're battling a disease, work with your doctor

178

to track exactly what's happening. for you. Is your tumor shrinking? Are your uterine fibroids disappearing? Is your heart rate coming back down into a healthy zone? If you struggle with a mental illness, like depression or an obsessive-compulsive disorder, are your symptoms lessening? Track things closely and see how things are progressing.

+ Look into the mirror. What do you notice? Is your skin clearing up? Does it seem smoother and softer, well-hydrated? Do your eyes seem brighter, more alert? Is your tongue bright and pink? Does your stomach look a little flatter, less puffy and bloated? All of these visual cues are great things to track, too.

+ Check in with yourself internally. How do you feel? Do you feel more optimistic? More energized? Are you sleeping more deeply? Do you wake up feeling activated instead of groggy? If you deal with anxiety, are your anxiety levels the same, or have they decreased?

+ Keep a written diary. Jot down a few sentences each day to record how you're feeling. Compare your entries from five weeks ago to today.

+ Keep a photo diary. Snap a selfie every day for five weeks. Try to stand in the same position (and the same lighting) each time. Compare your photos from five weeks ago to today. Notice any differences?

+ Notice how people react to you. I can't tell you how many times a client will visit me, and they'll say, "I just bumped into an old colleague from years ago. She didn't recognize me!" or "I just saw a photo of myself from a year ago. I barely recognized myself!" As your body detoxifies and heals, there are so many inner and outer changes that, yes, you might begin to look and feel like a different person. People might stop you and ask, "What have you been doing lately? You're glowing!" You can tell them, "I'm learning how to use food as healing medicine!" (And then offer to loan them this book!)

After the Five-Week Mark

Throughout this book, I've encouraged you to do a five-week challenge and follow the principles I've outlined for (at least) five weeks in a row. This will give your body a chance to flush out some toxins, soak in some nutrients, and begin all kinds of healing processes. Five weeks is usually long enough to notice some big changes.

So, what happens after the five-week mark? Great question.

At that point, I strongly encourage you to keep going... and going. Forever. Don't revert back to your old way of eating and living. Keep riding the wave of momentum you've created these last five weeks. Keep eating real food. Keep drinking nutrient-dense juices, at least one glass per day. Keep detoxifying your body with coffee enemas, keep on scraping your tongue, doing lymph massage and other gentle forms of detoxification. Keep taking your supplements, if you need them. You might not.

After five weeks, I have clients who tell me they want to incorporate a small amount of organic eggs, dairy, or even meat back into their diet. There's no dietary or nutritional reason to do so, but if you really feel you want to, then that's OK. Just make sure that your animal sources are clean and healthy. I have others who want to keep things strictly plant-based. That's OK, too. I have some clients who tell me they really miss pickles or kimchee, or healthy bread made with spelt, or some other specific type of food, and they want to add that back into their diet. That's fine.

I've noticed that most people want to maintain the positive changes they've made and want to stay completely away from heavily processed food.

"I feel so much better now, it's unbelievable," a client recently told me. "Putting crappy food into my body just isn't an option anymore."

Most of my clients just "feel different" about food. They tell me things like:

"I shop differently now. I really pay attention to where my food comes from."

"I've started going to the farmer's market with my kids every Saturday, and it's become one of our favorite family rituals."

"I used to eat so quickly, sitting in front of my computer or the TV, and now I've slowed down so much. I can actually taste my food. The whole experience feels so much better."

"I buy everything organic now. I used to think it didn't matter, but now I realize how much it does."

"I feel like I'm setting a better example for my kids. I know they're going to grow up with healthy eating habits, unlike I did. I feel proud that I'm creating a better future for them."

Who knows where you'll be, and what you'll feel like, five weeks from today? I'm excited for you to find out.

If you haven't started yet, start now. Even if it's 10:00 or 11:00 p.m., it's not too late to do something kind for your body today. Do five minutes of stretching. Make a glass of juice. Give yourself a massage to wake up your lymph system. Take ten minutes to chop some veggies for lunch tomorrow. You don't have to wait until tomorrow or next week or Monday to upgrade your life.

PART FOUR:

Your Whole Health Plan

Creating Your Whole Health Plan

We all know that cigarettes are toxic, but spending too many hours in your office chair? Just as bad. In fact, some researchers are saying that "sitting is the new smoking."

Most people here in North America sit at a desk for six to ten hours a day. As a culture, we've become incredibly sedentary, and this carries so many consequences for our health. A sedentary lifestyle is directly connected to chronic diseases like diabetes, cardiovascular disease, many types of cancer, and obesity.

And then, there's our stress levels. I feel stressed just thinking about stress!

This last year, in particular, I had to work really hard to keep my stress levels in check. Between running my two restaurant locations, opening six additional locations, preparing for a major TV appearance (competing on the reality TV show, *Dragon's Den*), creating this book plus a salad dressing cookbook, opening a brand-new wellness retreat center in British Columbia, giving my first TEDx talk, and managing the daily demands of being a wife and mom...whoa. It's been a wild ride.

I'm super-passionate about my work, which is a good thing, but too much of a good thing can be overwhelming. Like so many people, I have workaholic tendencies that I need to monitor closely and rein in.

So, why are we talking about sitting, smoking, and stress? Because for this final section of *Eat Real to Heal*, we're stepping outside of the kitchen. We're going beyond food. We're going to talk about the other components that make up a healthy lifestyle—your Whole Health Plan—which includes movement/exercise, stress-relief techniques, detoxifying your home environment, learning how to navigate the health care system as an informed, empowered, and savvy patient, and writing your own prescription for optimal health.

Yes, what you eat is important. I'd argue that changing your diet is the single most important change you can make. But there's a lot we need to consider, beyond food. So, let's dive in!

Movement

Our bodies were designed to move and move often. Personally, I know that I feel my best when I'm moving several times a week—walking, cycling, practicing yoga, hiking in the mountains with my family and our dog.

We all need to move. But we don't need to be fanatical about it. We live in a society where people often fall into extremes. On one side of the spectrum, we've got completely sedentary people who never, ever exercise. And on the other side, we've got CrossFit and Orange Theory devotees who put themselves through grueling workouts five to seven times a week, often without properly fueling their bodies, leading to exhaustion and injuries. There's a physical therapist based in the Pacific Northwest who has said, "I make a living thanks to CrossFit injuries. Thanks to CrossFit, I've got new clients arriving every day with sprained ankles, shoulder issues, you name it."

We need more balance.

There's a wonderful quote that's been floating around the internet for the last several years. It goes, "Exercise is not a punishment for what you ate. Exercise is a celebration of what your body can do."

It's true. If you're exercising fanatically because you want to burn eight hundred calories an hour to "make up for" the cheeseburger or brownies you had earlier, that's not a great situation. A much healthier mindset is to view exercise as a celebration of your wonderful, miraculous body, a celebration of being alive.

Exercise to stay fit and strong. Exercise to de-stress. Exercise to clear your mind. Exercise to spend time with friends. Exercise because it feels good. Exercise to celebrate this one precious body that you've got, not because you're trying to punish yourself.

You don't have to get yourself drenched in sweat for hours on end, and you don't need to push yourself to the brink of exhaustion. Keep it simple. Aim for moderation. And, if you're dealing with a disease like cancer, I strongly urge you to stop exercising for five weeks, at minimum, to give your body a chance to rest fully. Instead of hitting the gym, write a love letter to someone you care about, take a bath, get a massage, listen to music, or do some gentle stretching, but nothing too strenuous.

Once your body is fully healed, then yes, return to your regular exercise regime. But until then, I urge you to conserve your energy for healing, cellular regeneration, and detoxification.

I've had seriously sick clients—people dealing with cancer, for example—who really fight me on this. They tell me, "But I need to keep exercising! It's good for me!" Or they say, "Without daily exercise, I get really depressed." Here's something interesting: It's been shown that taking a twenty-minute walk in the woods is just as effective against depression as taking antidepressants or going for a one-hour run. So you can scale back your exercise regime and still get the mental/emotional benefits that you love.

Again, it's all about balance. Strike a balance that makes sense for your body, right now.

Managing Stress

Dr. Lissa Rankin is the author of a book called *Mind Over Medicine*. It's a wonderful book that describes how our lifestyle, including our mindset, directly impacts our health. I highly recommend that you check out this book, keep it on your bookshelf, and share it with your friends and family.

In her book, Rankin lays out a writing exercise you can do to identify the biggest sources of stress in your life and start to find some solutions. We're going to do a modified version of that exercise together, right now.

Grab a pen and paper.

Draw seven, eight, or maybe nine different circles on your piece of paper. As many as you want. They can all be different sizes. They don't need to be perfectly uniform. Just scribble like a kid.

Inside each circle, write down a particular area of your life:

1. Finances
2. Home
3. Career
4. Sexuality
5. My Partner/Spouse
6. Friends/Social Life

And then in those last couple of circles, write down any categories that come to mind. Maybe an area of your life that you've been worried about lately, or something you'd like to change or improve. It could be Style, Education, Community, Body Image, Food, Health, Creativity, Spirituality, or something else.

Spend some time looking at each circle, and thinking about each circle. Ask yourself, "How does this area of my life feel right now?" Next to each circle, mark down a number from one to ten. One means "Terrible." Ten means "Amazing."

For example, for Home, is your home decorated with furniture that you really love? When you step inside, does feel like a sanctuary? Or have you been following interior decor guidance from a magazine but somehow it never feels right, it doesn't feel like it's your space, and you never feel comfortable in it?

Rate all of your circles, one by one. Then make a list of the five categories that received the lowest scores. These are the five most stressful areas of your life.

I love this exercise because it identifies—usually, in just a matter of minutes—what's really stressing you out and weighing heavily on your body and mind. Sometimes, it's stuff we're not even aware of. I've done this exercise with hundreds of people over the last few years in workshop settings, and I'm always amazed by what comes out of it.

I've had people raise their hand and say, "I need to come out of the closet and be honest about my sexuality. I didn't realize how much stress all the secrecy has been causing me." I've had people announce to the room, "I need to leave my job. I'm ready to begin a new chapter doing something I love."

Testimonial

During one of our regular three-day retreats a few years ago, my guests completed this exercise and I gave everyone the opportunity to share their top stressor. Monica, an exuberant and confident middle-aged woman, shyly announced that she had always dreamed of leaving her long-time career as an accountant to become a painter. She felt stifled behind her desk, but sensed that she had a creative side that wanted out! Fast-forward two months and I found myself in a local art gallery in Whistler standing in front of a collection of deeply moving and colorful portraits of South American women engaged in a variety of different daily homesteading tasks. I was so captivated by the paintings that I didn't noticed that someone had walked up behind me and I jumped when the person asked, "Do you like these paintings?" I responded by saying, "Yes, so much so that I'm even considering buying one." I turned and looked up at the inquirer. Standing there was Monica with a proud and glowing smile on her face, and she announced that the stunning paintings that I was admiring were in fact hers.

By acknowledging one of her deepest stressors—lack of creativity in her life—Monica was then able to take action towards alleviating and shifting that stress. She told me that she was thriving once again and no longer felt stifled behind her desk in her daytime career, now that she had her creative outlet to inspire and motivate her.

When you can see your top five stressors written down, on paper, in your own handwriting, it's an eye-opening experience.

Now, you get to decide, "Which area will I tackle first? What's one thing I could do—this week—to improve the situation, and decrease my stress levels?" Then make a promise to yourself that you will take action to improving upon that situation, set a date, stick to it and get it done.

Enjoy this exercise. Teach it to your friends and family. Do it regularly—maybe once every six months, or once every year—just to check in again and identify stressors in your life.

I also encourage you to watch the TED Talk called "How To Make Stress Your Friend" by Kelly McGonigal. McGonigal's research shows that simply changing our perception of stress is enough to have a positive health impact. So even if you've got way too much going on in your life, if you view your stress load in a positive light, then it won't hinder your health as much. You can say to yourself, "Wow, I've got a ton of exciting projects at work right now! Lucky me!" rather than, "Aaaaaahhhhh, I've got so many projects at work right now. It's too much. I can't handle it." Simply changing the dialogue inside your mind can change your mood and also your physiology.

Unlimited Energy

Here's another mindset-shifting exercise that I love. Grab a fresh sheet of paper and a pen. Set a timer for ten minutes or put on a playlist that you love. Then write a few sentences about what you would do if you had unlimited amounts of energy.

What Would You Do with All of That Energy?

Would you open a business? Or a second business? Would you go cycling with your kids every day? Would you cook meals at home instead of ordering take-out? Would you lead an exciting community project? Would you have awesome sex every day? Would you hike more? Would you paint? Or write a book? Would you help your kids with their homework? Would you declutter your garage and transform it into a home-office sanctuary? Or something else?

I remember doing this exercise with a few people on a retreat, and it was so beautiful, because one of the men started to cry.

"The one thing I would do..." he said, "...is I would play with my kids more."

Often, we don't have enough energy to give others the love we want to give them—or receive the love we want to receive from others—because we're so exhausted.

Why are we exhausted? We're exhausted for so many different reasons: stress, the food we eat, a terrible night's sleep, the inundation of technology beeping and yapping at us all day long. Sometimes for eighteen hours a day. Sometimes, even in the middle of the night, when you're trying to get a good night's sleep, your phone goes off. We are inundated by so many things that are zapping our energy.

Once you've figured out what you would do if you had unlimited energy, then I challenge you to reclaim some of the energy you've lost. Take it back.

This could mean saying no to certain commitments you've kept in the past. It could mean upgrading your eating habits. It could mean prioritizing sleep. Or setting some new technology boundaries. Or setting new boundaries with clients, or with your boss. Whatever you need to do, just do it. This is your life. The only life you've got. Reclaim the energy you need to live, and thrive, and feel deep satisfaction.

Detoxifying the Home

Throughout this book, I've encouraged you to clean up your eating habits and switch to clean, organic, non-toxic food. Which is great. But for optimum health, you'll want to remove toxins from your home environment, too.

It seems kind of silly to eat plant-based food and do detoxifying enemas if your home is filled with toxic products, right? It's kind of like drinking a cold-pressed carrot juice and then drinking a Diet Dr. Pepper right afterward. You're pushing toxins out, and then pouring them right back in. We don't want that.

I vote, if you're going to detoxify, go ahead and detoxify everything you possibly can. Go all in!

The Kitchen

Let's start off with the kitchen. If you're using tablets or soap for the dishwasher, most likely, those products contain chlorine. The chlorine mixes with the hot water in the dishwasher and comes out as gas through the vents. This will fill your kitchen and home with chlorinated toxic air.

Of course, most of us think, "Well, it is just a little tiny bit. Besides, they wouldn't make that product if it wasn't safe."

Here's the thing. When cleaning products get tested to see if they are safe, most of the studies don't take into account that a person is usually exposed to an accumulation of different toxins—chlorinated dishwasher tablets, cosmetics, body and beauty products, sheets, pajamas, and carpets covered in fire retardant, lead paint in old buildings, asbestos, and so on.

Sure, maybe a little bit of chlorinated toxic air won't hurt you—but when it's combined with all the other toxins in your environment? Now it's not just a tiny drop. It's a tsunami! When these studies are being done, yes, they're testing the safe limit for one product—but they're not testing the safe limit for all of those products combined on a daily basis.

When I worked as an environmental consultant in Canadian government, we found that all of those toxins combined can wreak havoc on the human body. We now know that even one of those toxins in any area in your house can be enough to trigger mutation in our cells and get classified as a carcinogen. That's why I say, if there's anything you can detoxify in your home, do it. Every little change can make a difference.

Going back to the dishwasher—ditch those chlorinated tabs and switch to an all-natural product like borax (a.k.a sodium borate), baking soda, or white vinegar to rinse your dishes until they're sparkling clean. Google "non-toxic dishwasher fluid" or "non-toxic homemade dish cleaning solution" to find lots of options.

The Laundry Room

Bleach is not good for you. Inhaling bleach fumes can irritate the nose, eyes, skin, and lungs, and there's a correlation between bleach (which contains high amounts of chlorine) and cancer. I kicked the bleach habit a long time ago, and I've accepted that my clothes aren't always going to be pristine, bright, white, and that's okay with me. I'm fine with wearing a soft gray shirt that doesn't need bleach. I'd rather be healthy than have sparkling white tops.

Instead of using bleach, soak a soiled piece of clothing in a borax solution. Just dissolve a few small scoops of borax in some hot water and submerge your clothes. This will release most stains pretty nicely.

Also, ditch the dryer sheets. I never use them. They come with so many perfumes and dyes, and we just don't need all that crap coming into contact with our bodies. Plus, what do dryer sheets even do? I've never understood their purpose. Forget about 'em.

The Bathroom

Nobody wants to have a smelly toilet or dirty sink. We all want to have clean windows and mirrors in our bathroom. So, a lot of people use Windex—or similar products—to clear away the grime. Please do your body a favor and skip the electric blue, chemical-laden stuff. There are much safer, gentler alternatives. You can make a stellar cleaning spray using white vinegar, filtered water, and a few drops of aromatherapy essential oils, like rosemary or orange. And you can use baking soda to scrub grouts in between tiles.

My favorite product for cleaning the bathroom is called an "eco-cloth" or "magic cloth." It's fantastic! You can use it in your bathroom, kitchen, or all over your home for dusting. We use them for cleaning our windows. We always have two magic cloths for cleaning our windows—one dry and one wet.

The magic cloth is natural, it's built on the concept of Velcro. It has little tiny hooks in it which grab grease, dirt, and bacteria. It eliminates 99% of bacteria—just like bleach and other cleaning products do. You'll never need to have another spray bottle around. Simply take a wet cloth, wipe it down. Take the dry cloth, clean it up and you're done. Your windows are brilliant, sparkly and better cleaned than any other product I've ever found.

Also, do some decluttering inside your bathroom drawers and your shower. Are you one of the people who's got twenty different bottles of shampoo, conditioner, liquid soap, body scrubs, lotion, lip gloss, and other cosmetics? You really don't need all that stuff. Simplify and streamline. Choose a non-toxic, organic body wash like Dr. Bronner's soap. One bottle is highly concentrated and it will last for a surprisingly long time!

Always choose organic, non-toxic makeup if you want to wear cosmetics. One excellent brand is Dr. Hauschka (dr. hauschka.com), which was one of the first major cosmetics companies to offer cosmetics with minimally processed materials, straight from nature, no artificial colors, fragrances, or dyes, and no animal testing.

The Bedroom

Your bedroom should feel like a peaceful sanctuary. Unfortunately, many bedrooms contain all kinds of hidden toxins, especially in fabrics—sheets, pillows and clothing, and especially pajamas.

A lot of clothing companies use fire retardant materials, which are not safe for our body. It's important to buy clothes made of natural materials. Google "non-toxic pajamas" and you'll see a few brands to check out.

You can also switch to a non-toxic mattress. Think about it—you're pressed into your mattress for seven to nine hours, every single night. You're spending more time there than almost anywhere else! You want it to be non-toxic. My favorite mattress brand is the Sleep Natural, 100 percent organic natural latex mattress.

Finishing Touches

Go through your entire home, room by room, opening every cupboard and drawer. Don't forget your attic and all of those lawn and car products in your garage.

Toss anything that's expired and/or laden with chemicals into a trash bin. Give the house a nice, big cleaning session using safe products like borax, vinegar, lemon juice and baking soda. Start fresh.

Then, you can add a few finishing touches.

Make your own aromatherapy spray using water and a few drops of your favorite essential oil. Spritz your entire house. You can also get a vaporizer from a company like Saje and then you'll have lovely aromatherapy mist coming into your home, all the time, just like at a fancy spa.

I also recommend adding some living plants to every room. They look beautiful, and they also help to circulate oxygen more effectively throughout your home.

Then, beautify, adorn, and decorate your home with items that reinforce your commitment to leading a healthy lifestyle.

Maybe there are a couple of real food cookbooks that you love—put those on your kitchen table so they're in plain sight. Put your juicer in plain sight, too. Roll out a yoga mat. Put fresh flowers on your desk. Put a bowl of apples in the center of your kitchen. Tuck your smartphone in a drawer unless it's urgently needed. Adjust your environment so that it supports your new habits rather than hindering them. Set up your home so that it says, "A person who really cares about his/her health lives here."

Connecting with Nature

In the 1980s, researchers in Japan discovered something interesting about the connection between the human body and nature. Being in nature doesn't just "feel nice." It's actually a form of healing medicine for your body, and it has measurable effects.

Taking a stroll through a forest can lower your blood pressure, decrease your cortisol (stress hormone) levels, and boost the immune system by raising your lymphocyte count (lymphocytes are those courageous white blood cells that attack cancerous cells). Japanese researchers coined the term *Shinrin-yoku*, which means "forest bathing."

In a Shinrin-yoku study from 2007, men were instructed to take a two-hour walk in the woods. After just two walks (two days), their lymphocyte count went up by 50 percent, which means their bodies were better equipped to fight cancer and other diseases.

In 2008, a researcher named Dr. Li took a group of women on a three-day trip into nature. These women experienced profound physiological changes—including producing anti-cancer proteins—and the benefits lasted for more than seven days after the trip.

You can see more research at natureandforesttherapy.org and shinrin-yoku.org.

What's so exciting to me is that you don't need to spend thousands of hours in nature to reap these benefits. A few hours is enough. A stroll. A walk. A hike. A picnic. This is something that all of us can realistically do.

I love Richard Louv's book *Last Child in the Woods*,[7] which talks about the need for nature in our children's lives. But

---

7 http://richardlouv.com/books/last-child/

grown-ups need nature, too, not just kids. Think about the last time you spent a lovely day at the beach, or watched the sunset from your patio, or had lunch outside by a river, or visited a national park, or even a small neighborhood park. You probably felt steadier and calmer, like you could breathe more deeply, right? We all need, or can use, more nature connection in our lives.

Connecting to nature can be as simple as sitting on the sidewalk and taking time to just look, observe, and see a plant growing out from a crack on the sidewalk. It could mean packing your backpack and heading out to the woods for a three-day trek. You can do this with your loved ones or alone. Find out about the wonderful hikes in your community. You probably don't have to go too far. There will be hikes in your neighborhood and hikes right in your backyard, ranging into the mountain ranges, out onto the ocean, out onto the beaches, anywhere. Nature is all around us.

Another exciting trend is the "urban walk" phenomenon that's sweeping the world. In many big cities around the globe—like London and New York City—people are gathering to take a slow, mindful, tech-free walk through the city. No phones. No texting. No photos for Instagram. Just a lovely stroll through the city, stopping often to appreciate the trees, bushes, and flowers, as well as interesting historical and architectural details. Check out Urban Curiosity[8] to see a UK-based company that leads these kinds of walks. You could start an Urban Curiosity walking club in your city, too.

---

8 urbancuriosity.co.uk

Become a Tree-Hugger

The act of placing your hand on a tree trunk, or even wrapping your arms around the tree, has been proven to shift our bodies on a physiological level. It reduces blood pressure, has a positive effect on cholesterol, and can even alleviate symptoms of depression.

Researchers who study depression have found that there's no antidepressant medication out there that has a better effect than exercise, being in nature, and moving our bodies.

If you suffer from depression, or even if you're just having a sluggish, gloomy day, step outside in bare feet and let your skin come into direct contact with the earth. Feel the grass, the soil, the sand. Be there. Breathe it in. Find a nearby tree, if possible. Press your palms into the tree or wrap your arms around it. Imagine light, love, and calmness flooding from the tree into your own body. Imagine yourself plugging into a natural battery, soaking in powerful healing energy, recharging your immune system.

This may sound like a "hippie" thing to do, or just "silly" or even "crazy," but the research doesn't lie. We know, without a doubt, that connecting with nature has a direct impact on what's happening inside your body. It's not silly. It's powerful.

I encourage you to connect with nature at least once or twice this week. Write down the locations you want to go, places that inspire you. Maybe you even want to save up for a trip to an amazing location somewhere in the world?

And if you hug a tree sometime this week, please email me and my team and tell us how it felt.[9] We'd love to hear your story. And we bet that tree loved hugging you back.

---

[9] info@richerhealthretreatcentre.com

Connecting with Your Breath

Breathing. It is the very first thing we do when we enter this world. It is the last thing we do before we pass away and move out of this world. It is the pulse of life.

Over fourteen years ago, I was certified as a yoga instructor. In yoga, the number-one thing I would always focus on when teaching is breathing. I'd tell my students, "Remember your breath." "Don't forget to breathe." "Keep breathing"…over and over. I didn't care if my students could do the poses "perfectly" or if they looked like super bendy-stretchy models from the cover of *Yoga Journal*. That doesn't matter! What matters is that you keep breathing throughout the class, because that's how you'll receive the health benefits of practicing yoga.

If you look at a baby or small child, they know how to breathe deeply and fully. They take beautiful, deep breaths in and out, all day long. You can see their bellies inflate and deflate with each breath.

Now, compare that to how most adults breathe. If you say to a grown-up, "Take a big, deep breath," what happens? You'll see their shoulders scrunch up, their neck become strained, their chest might inflate a bit. They're breathing in a tight, shallow way, high up in the chest—not breathing deeply and easily like we all used to do as children. Most grown-ups need to "re-learn" how to breathe deeply. Fortunately, it's not hard to do. Here are some exercises you can try.

Simple Breathing Exercises

In the Morning

First thing in the morning, when you wake up, roll onto your back, stare up at the ceiling, place a hand on your belly, and just allow the breath to move into that part of your body. Let your belly expand upward and downwards. Imagine this pure, energizing breath filling up your chest cavity, your belly, and moving down your legs, down your arms, and out your fingertips. Visualize breath and life moving into all parts of your body.

Any Time of Day

Here's another breathing exercise that's really simple: place one hand on your belly, invite breath into your body and count to five. Inhale for 1, 2, 3, 4, 5. Hold the breath for two counts. Next, exhale for twice the counts you inhaled. Exhale for 1, 2, 3, 4, 5, 6, 7, 8, 9, 10, until your hand compresses your belly. Breathe in again for five counts, then draw your belly button back toward your spine and let out every last drop of breath in your body for ten counts.

Then repeat. Inhale for five. Exhale for ten. Inhale. Exhale. Keep repeating for a few minutes. If you're ever feeling shaky, anxious, worried, or distracted, this is a fast way to quiet down your mind. It's so good for your circulatory system, your immune system, all the beautiful systems in your body.

If you start off doing this and you can't exhale for the full count of ten, no problem. Inhale for a count of three and exhale for a count of six. Or inhale for a count of four and exhale for a count of eight. The important thing is that your exhalation is slower and longer than your inhalation.

When You're Feeling Sluggish, Tired, or Cold

Have you ever tried alternate-nostril breathing, or *Nadi*

Shodhana? This is an effective breathing technique to balance the brain and quiet and focus the mind. It's one of my favorite breathing techniques to teach during yoga classes. In the Kundalini yoga tradition, I also like what's called the "skull shining breath," the "fire breathing" exercise, or sometimes "breath of fire."

This type of breath creates heat in the body. You can do this to wake up your body before a workout, to build energy if you're feeling sluggish, or to warm yourself up on a chilly winter morning.

I'll guide you through the alternate-nostril breathing exercise, coupled with the fire breathing exercise. If you are interested in learning more about each individual breathing technique, you can simply Google YouTube videos about the "skull shining breath" or "*Kapalabhati* breathing" or *Nadi Shodhana*, or the alternate-nostril breathing technique. They are all fantastic body healing breathing exercises. Try them all.

Sit comfortably with a tall, straight spine. Place your right thumb over your right nostril and press gently to seal it closed. Now, inhale and exhale through your left nostril only. Start at a normal pace. Then quicken things up. Inhale and exhale quickly through your left nostril ten to twenty times in a row. Exhale forcefully, like you want to puff air out of your nostril with intensity. With each exhale, you should feel your belly muscles contract in, just a tiny bit.

After ten to twenty times, switch sides. Plug your left nostril with your left thumb. Inhale and exhale quickly through your right nostril, ten to twenty times. Repeat this cycle a few times. You'll notice heat building in your body. You might feel more clear-headed and awake.

If you start feeling dizzy or light-headed, just slow down your breathing pace a bit.

Those are just a couple of breathing techniques you can try. I invite you to Google "Yoga breathing exercise" or "Stress relief with breathing" to find dozens of other techniques.

The simple act of taking one big, deep breath can change your physiology instantly. Your heart rate decelerates. Your shoulders relax. It's such a gift for your body, and—unlike taking prescription meds—breathing is free, instant, and there are zero negative side effects.

Hydration and Water Contamination

The human body is made up of 70 to 90 percent water. It's no secret that we need water to survive. When we're dehydrated, all kinds of problems occur. Headaches. Dry skin. Dizziness. Fever. Dangerously low blood pressure. Seizures. Comas. Even death.

You might think, "Well, I don't feel any of those symptoms, so I'm probably doing fine." But that may or may not be true. You might be dehydrated on an organ and tissue and cellular level even if you don't feel thirsty. Even worse, you might be drinking water that is severely contaminated.

To avoid drinking contaminated water, consider drinking nutrient-dense cold-pressed organic juices!

What's Actually In Your Water?

I live in Whistler, British Columbia—a region that's known for its pristine mountains and skiing slopes, natural beauty, and crisp air. The air smells clean. Everything looks clean. You get water from the tap and it tastes pretty clean, too. But appearances can be deceiving. In reality, there are a lot of unhealthy contaminants and chemicals in the water, even in a gorgeous place like Whistler.

Think about the journey water takes from its origin to your faucet at home. Water goes from the clouds to lakes and rivers, and then it's captured somewhere, usually in a man-made reservoir.

In that reservoir, in most parts of the world, water gets treated to remove harmful bacteria, parasites, etc. Chemicals like chlorine, fluorosilicic acid, aluminum sulfate, and many others get pumped into the water. OK, the bad bacteria get eliminated—that's good. But there's an unwanted consequence, because now the water is filled with chemicals that are linked to cancer and other chronic diseases.

Then the water flows through underground pipes which carry it through the city into your home. Often, these pipes are fifty, seventy, even one hundred years old or more. In some cities, the pipes were built in the Victorian era! These old pipes often contain traces of all kinds of toxic substances, like arsenic, radium, and mercury. As it passes through, your drinking water picks up all of these substances—not to mention pesticides, the commonly used agricultural herbicide, glyphosate, and other toxins that seep down through the soil, yikes.

By the time that water gets to your kitchen faucet, it's often full of dozens of substances that you definitely *do not* want inside your body.

You can purchase a drinking-water test kit online at Amazon.com for less than twenty dollars. This is a quick way to test your water for chlorine, pesticides, and other toxins, and see what's actually in your drinking water. You might be shocked.

"But, wait a minute, if our water is really so terrible, wouldn't the government intervene and fix it?" you might be wondering. "Surely they wouldn't let everyone drink unhealthy water?"

Yes, it is our local government's job to keep our water safe and clean. They do their best. But it's usually not enough, as they are working hard to meet the minimum standards for community health. Also, there's huge disagreement about what's considered safe and what's not. Sometimes scientists still insist that chlorine is fine, for example, while others insist that it's undeniably linked to cancer.

We Can't Sit Back and Wait

Are we going to wait for scientists to finish arguing about water safety and come to a consensus? Are we going to wait around for science to catch up with reality? Are we going to wait and wait, while toxicity accumulates in our systems with every glass of water we drink?

In my opinion, we can't afford to sit back and wait. We can't place our health in other people's hands and trust that everything is safe and fine. We have to take personal responsibility for our bodies.

Let's not forget...there was a time in human history, not too long ago, when people believed the earth was flat. They were wrong. There was time when scientists believed that cigarettes were good for you, that they could protect your throat, and help you live longer. They were wrong. About one hundred years ago, many physicians thought that cocaine was a great remedy for seasonal allergies. They were wrong. There are so many instances throughout history where the "experts" insist that something is safe, even healthy, and they're dead wrong.

My point is, we have to question authority. We can't blindly accept what we're told, or what's advertised in magazines, or blindly trust the latest government statement that insists our water is fine. We need to proceed with a healthy degree of skepticism, and we have to take matters into our own hands.

One of the simplest ways to do this is to get a water filtration system for your home.

My Favorite Water Filtration Systems

You can get a Brita filter,[10] or a similar product. Those are inexpensive and work OK. However, my personal favorite is the Berkey water filter (berkeyfilters.com). It's incredible. It catches 99 percent of contaminants while preserving the good minerals that you want. When there's a military or environmental disaster somewhere in the world, the Berkey filter is THE filter of choice that's shipped to that region. With a Berkey, you can scoop water from a river, lake, even a swamp or a puddle, put it into this filter, and you're left with beautiful, clean water.

You can also invest in a water distiller, which can run about $200. Typically, these devices sit on your countertop. They use heat to separate water from chemicals and other minerals. They're very powerful. For a few hundred dollars, you're making an investment than can lengthen your lifespan.

But our drinking water is just the beginning. We also need to consider the water that we splash onto our faces in the sink, and the water in our showers and bathtubs. After all, your skin is the largest organ of your body. Water gets absorbed into your skin every day. You want that water to be pure and uncontaminated. That's why I highly recommend getting a filtration system for your shower, too. You can get one that's small and easy to attach. Google "shower water filtration system" to see your options. This is another small, simple, affordable way to take your health back into your own hands.

We can't always directly control the government's decisions, or what's happening in the power plant on the edge of town, or what's seeping into the city reservoir. But at least we can control what's happening inside our own homes. To me, this is very exciting. Instead of feeling hopeless and powerless, we can take back our power.

---

10 brita.com

Goals and Your Subconscious Mind

Has this ever happened to you?

You set a big, beautiful goal for yourself. Maybe you want to ditch junk food and switch to real, organic food. Maybe you want to practice yoga every day. Or write a book. Or watch less TV and spend more time outside. Or wipe out your credit-card debt.

You set the goal. You start working on it. But pretty soon—after a few weeks, days, or even just a few hours— something blocks you. You start feeling anxious, tired, or overwhelmed. Or maybe you're not sure what you're feeling, exactly. But something is impeding your progress. It's like you're moving through sticky ice-cold molasses instead of fresh air. It just feels so...hard! Before you know it, you're diving into a plate of deep-fried onion rings or buying a $500 purse that you can't really afford, even though that's the opposite of your goal! But why is this happening?!

It's so frustrating, right? You want something. You set a goal. Why can't you just DO IT?

If you struggle to achieve your goals—and believe me, most people do—one of the best techniques I've ever studied combines the use of your mind and your body.

With this technique, you explore how it will feel to achieve this goal. You look at the rewards and also the adverse consequences of achieving this goal. You dig into your subconscious mind to discover what's really stopping you from pursuing this goal. The answer might surprise you. Often, it's not what we expect.

I've explored numerous techniques for achieving goals— and transforming daily habits—over the years. Out of everything I've studied, I've found this technique to be the most effective. If you're curious to try it out, here's an exercise you can do right now...

Mind-Body Balance Exercise

Set aside twenty to thirty minutes to do this exercise. There are a couple of parts, and you want to feel relaxed, not pressured and rushed.

Get a pen and some paper. Think about a goal that you want to achieve. It can be a health and wellness-related goal, a professional goal, a personal goal, anything that feels important to you. Write this goal down. But as you're writing it down, hold these five principles in mind:

1. **Write down your goal "as if" you already have it**
   Instead of writing: *I would like to adopt a cute Golden Retriever puppy*, you would write: *I have a cute Golden Retriever puppy.* Write down your goal as if you've already achieved it, as if it's already happening in your life. By doing this, you are rewiring your brain to invite this new reality into your life.

2. **Keep it short and sweet.** You don't want to have a goal that is confusing and long-winded. For example: *I have unlimited health, wealth, happiness, and I've got the perfect job of my dreams, and a partner who adores me.* This is too long. Keep it shorter.

3. **Be as specific as you can.** You might write down a goal that says: *I have unlimited wealth.* That's a great goal. However, let's get even more specific. One time, I wrote down the following goal: *I easily maintain $30,000 in my bank account at all times.* Do you see how the second goal is highly specific? The more specific you can be, the better.

4. **Choose a goal that's emotionally charged.** Maybe you write down a goal like: *I do Pilates every day for thirty minutes.* You read it back and you think, "OK,

206

yeah, that sounds nice, sure." But you don't feel any emotion. You're not fired up and excited about it. Guess what? That's probably not a goal you should pursue, because deep down, it's just not a true priority for you.

Next, maybe you write down: *I play with my daughter every night before bedtime,* or *We read a story together every night.* This time, you read the goal and you feel teary-eyed and emotional. This time, you've written down a goal that really matters to you.

When you're setting goals in life, you want to pick goals that get you all fired-up inside, that give you shivers, and make you almost want to cry, laugh, scream, or say "Yes! This is the one." If you're emotionally charged-up, then you're way more likely to take this goal seriously and really make it happen.

5. **Keep it positive.** Here's an example: *I don't want to be poor.* That's a great goal. However, it's written in a negative way. It's important that you shuffle the wording around. The new, adjusted goal can be: *I pay my bills on time every month,* or *I have $20,000 in my savings account.* Instead of: *I don't want to be sick,* flip it to: *I feel strong and vibrant.* Instead of: *I don't want to be alone,* that goal can become: *I am surrounded by supportive friends, family, and a stellar Whole Health Team.*

Write down your goal using these five principles to guide you.

Next, I want you to ask yourself:

"What Are Three Specific Things That Would Indicate I've Achieved This Goal?"

For example, if your goal is: *I have my dream job,* what would that look like? What are three things that might be in your office that would indicate—to an outside observer, looking in—that you've done it? What are three specific, tangible markers of success?

For you, it might be:

1. There's a $5,000 check from a client sitting on my desk.

2. There's a three-week vacation booked on my calendar, because my dream job includes plenty of space for rest and recharging.

3. There's a plane ticket to NYC on my desk because I've been invited to speak at a conference there.

4. Try this with your goal. Whatever kind of goal you wrote down, come up with three specific, visible, tangible things that would indicate that you're "there" or you've "done it."

What would be in your home? On your desk? On your calendar? In your inbox? Hanging in your closet? What colors have you painted your walls? What's the exact number in your bank account? Come up with a couple ideas.

Below that, write down how you're going to feel once you achieve this goal. Are you going to feel proud? Energized? Awake? Alive? Connected? Supported? Write down a few words that sums up how you'll feel.

Then, close your eyes, and try to remember a time in your life when you felt this same feeling. A memory. A moment. Let it wash over you. Sink into that feeling. Feel your entire body filling up completely with this feeling. When you think about the color of that feeling, what would it be? What would the temperature be? What would the texture and shape of that feeling be? What does it look like? Where do you feel it inside your body? Really connect with this feeling.

When you're ready, open your eyes. At this point, you've established a specific goal. You've figured out three markers of success that will indicate you've achieved this goal. You've realized how it will feel once you do. The next part of this exercise gets a little bit trickier. Now, I invite you to think about the adverse consequences of achieving your goal.

Most people think, "That's crazy. Why would there be any adverse consequences? It is going to be fantastic." Yes, it's going to be fantastic. However, to achieve something new, we must give up something old. There's always a trade-off.

Here's an example:

Let's say I want to lose twenty pounds, become physically fit, and complete a marathon. To achieve this goal, I will need to train regularly. I will need to change my diet to make sure I'm flooding my body with plenty of nutrients. I will need to go to bed earlier and rest more so that my body can recover from intense workouts, which means I miss out on other things that I enjoy. I may have to give up time with friends and family in order to exercise. I may have to wear Spandex running clothes I don't like. I may have to spend money on specific classes, tools, equipment, and training. I may have to hire somebody to tell me what to do, like a coach or trainer. Maybe I don't enjoy being told what to do! All the things I just listed might be considered adverse consequences.

Sometimes, our subconscious mind gets anxious about these adverse consequences and decides, "I don't like the sound of that. No way. I'm going to block [your name here] from pursuing this goal." Then what happens? You start sabotaging yourself. You struggle to move forward with your goal, almost as if you're locked in a battle with your own mind. Because, quite literally, you are!

Once I had a client who'd been diagnosed with a debilitating disease. She told me, "I want to beat this disease. I want to feel better." I worked with her closely, teaching her how to upgrade her eating habits and lifestyle, how to detoxify her system, all the things we've covered in this book. She promised she would do everything. And did she? No. In fact, she barely implemented any of the changes we discussed.

During a follow-up session, she felt ashamed, almost on the brink of tears. "Nicolette," she told me. "I swear I want to get better. But, for some reason, I feel so blocked. I want to change my lifestyle, but somehow I can't seem to get started."

We did this exercise together. When we got to the part about adverse consequences, we uncorked some interesting information. As an adverse consequence, my client wrote down: *I'd have to return back to my normal life.*

My client had been seriously ill for a long time. As a result, she didn't have a full-time job. She didn't have to pay rent or a mortgage. While she didn't enjoy being sick, on some level, she enjoyed the freedom and overall lack of responsibilities that being sick provided. She was reluctant to give that up. She wanted to be healthy, of course—but to do that, there would be a trade-off. Was she willing to make the trade?

Are you?

This is a big question. I invite you to sit with it, as long as you need. Consider your goal. Consider the benefits that you'll get. Consider the adverse consequences, too—the trade-off, the sacrifice. Consider if the sacrifice will be worth it. Will it? Only you can answer that question for yourself.

Ultimately, if you choose to proceed with this goal, you want to proceed with your whole heart, mind, and body on board. This means fully understanding the goal from all angles—the rewards and also the sacrifices—and making a fully informed decision.

Lastly, here's how you can seal this goal into your heart, mind, and body, and make the commitment official.

Go into a private space, like your bedroom. Close the door if you need additional privacy. Sit in a chair or the edge of your bed. Sit comfortably with a tall, straight spine.

Hold your arms in front of you. Cross your right arm over your left. Rotate your palms so that your thumbs are facing down, palms facing each other. Clasp your hands gently together. Then bend your elbows and bring your clasped hands towards your heart, almost like a prayer position. Cross your ankles. This is a calming posture that encourages your parasympathetic nervous system to settle down. It's excellent for reducing anxiety. Then close your eyes.

As your eyes are closed, seated in this position, repeat your goal to yourself. Say it quietly, to yourself, in your head, over and over. Remember to speak in the present tense, as if you already have achieved this goal.

Say: *I easily maintain $30,000 in my bank account at all times.*

Or say: *I play with my daughter every night before bedtime.*

Or: *I have reversed my diabetes and I am healthy, fit, and disease-free.*

Keep repeating your goal aloud, over and over, until you feel a shift in your body. This shift might feel like hiccups, laughter, crying, a big release of tension in your shoulders, a feeling of clarity and lightness in your body, or maybe something else. When it happens, you will know. When this shift occurs—it might be a spiritual, physical, emotional, or mental shift—that signals that something has shifted in your subconscious mind. Some type of block has been dissolved. Now, achieving your goal will be easier. Not "easy," necessarily. But much easier. You've removed some of the impediments in your way.

Once this shift occurs, open your eyes, and say:

I am ready to welcome this goal into my life!

Yes, you are!

You can do this exercise whenever you want to set a new goal or commit more strongly to a goal you've already set. I do this exercise all the time with my children. They often run up to me and say: "Mom, can you balance me for this? Can you balance for that?" It's a beautiful way of getting in touch with your goals, visualizing and experiencing what that goal is going to be like, and setting yourself up for success.

When you do this exercise, you're inviting your subconscious mind to work with you, rather than sabotaging you.

It's like having a meeting with your team at work and saying, "OK, does everybody understand our mission? Does everyone understand the sacrifices that will need to be made, and also the amazing rewards that are waiting ahead? Is everyone on board, ready to work towards the goal?" You want everyone on your team to say, "Yes!"

It's the same with your mind. You want all parts of your mind—your conscious mind and your subconscious mind— to work together towards a shared goal. You don't want a fragmented mind that's full of disagreement. You want a unified mind. Using techniques like this can shift your mind into this place and help you achieve anything you want, even goals you've neglected or struggled with before. Try it and see.

Becoming a Savvy Patient

As human beings, we are taught from a very early age to trust in authority figures. "Don't talk to strangers," your parents probably told you, as well as, "Listen to your teacher," and "Do what the doctor says."

We grow up this way. As adults, we're hardwired to trust people in positions of authority. We see a white lab coat and we immediately think, "I should do whatever this person tells me."

One researcher did an experiment[11] where they had doctors wear white lab coats, scrubs, professional office attire, and then casual attire. The researchers found that people immediately trusted the doctors more if they wore a white lab coat. The white lab coat scored about 76 percent for trust and confidence. Scrubs got about 10 percent. Casual attire got just 4 percent . Same doctor. Different outfits. Different reactions.

As this experiment shows, we make split-second decisions about the people we meet. A police uniform, a blazer and pantsuit, a white lab coat—these are cultural, visual cues that lead us to think, "I should do whatever this person says."

But blind obedience isn't a good thing—especially when it comes to our health.

All too often, we "follow the doctor's orders" even when our instincts tell us to do otherwise. I can't tell you how many people have come to me over the years, each telling me some version of the same story:

"I felt like something was wrong. But my doctor told me everything was fine. For years and years, they told me there was nothing wrong. Then last week I found out I have cancer, and it's stage IV."

I've heard this story countless times. Not just with cancer, but with all kinds of diseases.

---

11 http://www.amjmed.com/article/S0002-9343(05)00351-7/abstract

The moral of the story? Your doctor may be very well-educated, very wise, very loving, very caring, and very good at his or her job. But that doesn't mean you should believe everything she says or do everything she recommends.

Doctors are not infallible. Doctors make mistakes. That's why it's crucial to become a savvy patient and take ownership of your health. This means trusting your instincts, questioning authority, and also building a Whole Health Team that includes numerous people, not just one. You want a variety of perspectives and healing modalities, not just one person's opinion.

The Power of a Whole Health Team

Why put together a Whole Health Team? Why have multiple healers working together, instead of just your regular doc? Here's a story from my own life that illustrates the power of collaboration.

When my daughter was nine years old, she was goofing around with some friends, doing upside-down yoga poses in an aerial yoga swing.

She climbed up about eight feet, but then she lost her balance, flipped over, and smacked her head on the ground. Fortunately, she didn't have any broken bones, but she did end up with a severe concussion.

If any of you have experienced a bad concussion, you know how debilitating it can be. My daughter's head was throbbing. The pain was so intense. She couldn't play. She couldn't go to school. Her vision was impaired. She couldn't sleep properly. Her mood was completely different. She wasn't herself. It was really scary.

This went on for thirty days. She wasn't improving. The pain remained very intense. I took her back to the doctor several times, and eventually the doctor told me there was nothing more they could do. He also told me it could take a year or longer for my daughter to heal.

He told me she'd probably need to be out of school for...
a year.

A year?! Can you believe that? As a mom, I thought to
myself, "OK, that's ridiculous. That can't be the final answer.
There's got to be *something* we could do to help her."

I felt really discouraged by this doctor's pessimistic attitude.
I decided, "I can't accept this. I am going to take matters
into my own hands."

What happened next? I assembled the best team I could
put together. I found a physiotherapist, an acupuncture
practitioner, an optometrist, a magnesium float-tank
business, intense neuro-nutrition, compression therapy,
and a chiropractor. I decided we were going to try every
possible solution to help my daughter feel better. I put
together a powerhouse healing team and plan, and I
executed that plan in one day.

The optometrist suggested putting tape over the sides of
my daughter's glasses to block her peripheral vision.
If she's getting fewer visual stimuli, it might reduce the pain.
We tried that, and it worked! Her pain levels decreased.
Incredible. Such a simple thing, and it made such a
difference. The physio appointment followed immediately by
acupuncture also brought her pain levels down.

I knew through my research about stress and injury that
magnesium is a potent and necessary mineral for repair and
regeneration, so I brought my daughter to a local business
that offers magnesium therapy float tanks. My daughter
soaked and rested in the magnesium bath for ninety
minutes. Again, her pain decreased. After a concussion,
the body typically suffers some magnesium loss, so doing
magnesium baths can help to replenish the levels.

After that busy morning, I fed my daughter a nutrient-dense

brain-health meal (and a veggie juice of course), and then I applied compression therapy to her entire body. She fell into a deep and restful sleep for over two hours. This was the first nap she'd taken since she was three years old and the first deep sleep she had experienced since she received the concussion. When she woke up, her pain levels were down to a one out of ten. It was obvious that she felt so much better. I could see the sparkle coming back into her eyes.

After more nutrient-rich brain food full of omega-3s, I took her to our local and trusted chiropractor who did several adjustments and brought her skeletal system back into full alignment. After that, her pain was gone. Entirely. In just one day. And she returned to school the very next day and didn't miss a day of school afterward as a result of that concussion.

Again, that first doctor told me that my daughter would be out of school for *an entire year*. But once we got a multi-faceted healing team together, it only took *one day* to bring her pain levels from a ten out of ten down to a zero and bring her completely back to normal. The next day, she was back at school with no pain, totally back to her usual routine and her joyful quirky self. What a relief.

This experience reminded me that getting one physician's opinion is *not enough*. In fact, in some instances, trusting one physician's recommendation can be *disastrous*.

Can you imagine if I'd believed that first doctor? Can you imagine if I'd pulled my daughter out of school for one year, as he recommended? That's something that would have negatively impacted her entire childhood, and possibly her entire life.

I'm so grateful that I listened to my instincts and acted like a savvy patient, rather than a passive patient. By putting together a Whole Health Team, we eradicated my daughter's pain and got her life back on track.

In our current system, you go see a doctor, you spend seven and a half minutes together (if you're fortunate enough to get that much time), they make a diagnosis, and they usually prescribe some medication, because that's what they're trained to do. Or, if there's no medication that can be prescribed, then you're often told, "Sorry, there's nothing we can do. Just rest and let's see what happens."

I'm sorry, but that's just not good enough. We deserve much better care than that. We need teams of healers working together, communicating together, and using every possible healing modality to help people get better. Building this team starts with *you*. You have to seek it out, demand it, and build it yourself.

Ask the Right Questions

To be a savvy patient and build a Whole Health Team, first, you need to fully understand your diagnosis. You need to collect all the facts. This means asking lots and lots of questions.

If you've been diagnosed with a particular type of cancer, for example, you'll want to ask your doctor questions like:

+ How many people live when they do absolutely nothing after they've been diagnosed?

+ How long do people with the exact same diagnosis live if they choose to do chemo, surgery, radiation, or another type of medical treatment?

+ How many people live if they skip chemo and choose to do an alternative or complementary therapy like the Gerson Therapy, the Budwig Diet, or something else?

Those are key questions to ask. It's really important that your oncologist or medical doctor can answer those questions, because that's the information that will help you make an informed decision about what to do next.

You can ask similar questions for any kind of condition. Say, migraines. When you're given a prescription drug for migraines, ask your doctor:

+ What are the side effects?

+ How effective is this drug? Is it likely to relieve symptoms by 50 percent? 100 percent?

+ How long will I need to take it?

+ Will I need to increase the dosage over time?

+ If my body gets used to taking this drug, will I need to switch drugs in the future?

Another question I like to ask is:

+ How do you know it's not X, Y, or Z?

By asking this, you're encouraging your doctor to think more expansively and get into a different frame of thinking.

Here's an example: When one of my daughters was eight years old, we brought her in to the doctor because she had a cold, or possibly a flu bug. She was feverish, had a headache, and felt tired, along with a few other symptoms. It seemed like a common cold. But I had a feeling there was something else going on.

Sure enough, the doctor said: "She has a cold. Take her home and give her liquids, plenty of rest, and monitor her health."

I took her home. But instinctively, as her mother, I knew that something else was up. That night, I listened to her breathing and I heard some gurgling in her chest— which may mean pneumonia, or possibly something even more severe.

I brought her back to the doctor's office the next day and demanded a test for pneumonia, including X-rays. The doctor thought I was overreacting and didn't want to do these tests. They probably thought I was a hypochondriac mother who spent too much time on Google researching symptoms. But I insisted.

With a firm tone of voice, I asked the doctor, "OK, you're pretty certain she's got a cold. It might be a cold. But how do you know it's not pneumonia? How do you know it's not meningitis? Are you completely sure?"

My doctor agreed that, yes, it's possible it could be something else. He agreed to run more tests. Long story short, after several tests, and four days of waiting for test results, the news came back: it was meningitis.

Meningitis is a serious disease that often mimics flu symptoms, but it's far more severe. Left untreated, it can lead to permanent brain damage, seizures, hearing loss, even death. Can you imagine if I'd trusted the doctor's assessment ("It's just a cold") instead of listening to my intuition? My daughter could be dead right now. This may sound dramatic, but that's the reality.

Yes, your doctor went to medical school for six to ten years. Yes, your doctor is thoughtful, careful, and wants only the best for you. Even so, we can't ever place our health—our lives—into the hands of just one person. At the end of the day, these doctors are just human beings, and human beings make mistakes all the time. It's crucial to ask questions, and then ask follow-up questions, and advocate for your own health.

The Facts about Medical Error

Here in North America, today, the number-one cause of death is cancer. The number-two cause of death is heart disease. Can you guess the third leading cause of death?

You might guess complications related to diabetes, or obesity, or perhaps suicide. No. Research shows that the third leading cause of death is *medical error.*

What does a medical error look like? It can mean taking a prescription medication that interacts badly with another medication, resulting in death. It can mean putting the wrong pills into a bottle that's labeled with a totally different kind of medication—which happens in pharmacies more often than you'd think. It can mean doing surgery on the wrong organ or limb—this, too, happens more often than you think. Another form of medical error is when a medical practitioner doesn't diagnose someone correctly. Then that person leaves the office or hospital and experiences life-altering consequences because of getting the wrong diagnosis.

It's been reported that 10–20 percent of patients are misdiagnosed, and 28 percent of misdiagnosed patients wind up dead or permanently disabled. This is a huge issue in the medical field, and one that's rarely discussed.

Again, I have the utmost respect for doctors. But at the end of the day, we're all human. Nobody is correct 100 percent of the time. This is why, as a savvy patient, you need to trust your intuition and push for extra medical tests if you feel you've been misdiagnosed. Don't worry about seeming "bossy" or "pushy" or too "demanding." This is your life we're talking about. It's not to be taken lightly. Push for the best possible care. Don't settle for anything less.

Now that you know the third leading cause of death in North America is medical error, what are you going to do about it?

For starters, take a closer look at the medications you're currently taking—if you're taking any. Go online and research them. Look at the pamphlet that the pharmacist hand to you. Triple-check to make sure this drug won't negatively interact with any other drugs that you're taking, or with food that you're eating.

For example, some antibiotics can reduce the effectiveness of your oral birth control pills—if you don't want to get pregnant, that's a pretty important detail to know about! Combining antidepressants like Zoloft with methadone can have fatal consequences. Eating grapefruit while taking statins (to control cholesterol) or many other drugs can have adverse effects. There are so many interactions and combinations that you need to be fully aware of.

Most people never even open up these drug pamphlets, and most people don't bother to read the "fine print" because they assume, "My doctor told me to take this, so it's fine." This might not be the case. You need to double— and triple—check the details.

I highly encourage you to read Dr. Carolyn Dean's book *Death by Modern Medicine*.[12] Read that book from start to finish. It highlights some of the drugs on the market that really should not be prescribed because the side effects are so severe.

What else can you do to be a savvy patient? A lot! You can even call lawyers' offices to get the full scoop on what's happening with drugs like Vioxx. This is a drug that's often prescribed for illnesses like arthritis. It has been banned in other countries—but not in North America—even though we know it's causing thousands of deaths a year. Your doctor might not say this to you. It's up to you to be a savvy patient and dig up the truth.

Google the drugs that have been recommended to you. Research thoroughly. Consider the pros and cons. Consider your alternative options. Ask questions—lots of questions— and don't allow your doctor (or anybody else on your team) to brush you off dismissively.

---

12 http://www.drcarolyndean.com/content/?section=death_by_modern_medicine&page=details

Again, *this is your life.*

If you struggle to stand up for yourself, if you feel intimidated by authority figures, then pretend that you're advocating for your child, for your partner, for someone you love fiercely.

Imagine your doctor gives your child a diagnosis and you suspect it's not right. What would you do? Hopefully, you would push back, you would dig deeper, you would do anything and everything to heal your child, right? You would become a health warrior. You would fight fiercely and relentlessly.

The same way you'd behave if your child was in potential danger—that's how you need to behave when it comes to your own health, too.

Build Your Whole Health Team

Who needs to be on your Whole Health Team? The answer to that question is different for everyone, of course. Your team might include:

+ Your general physician
+ An endocrinologist
+ An oncologist
+ A physiotherapist
+ A massage therapist
+ A chiropractor
+ An acupuncturist
+ An Ayurvedic practitioner
+ A Chinese medicine practitioner
+ A Reiki practitioner
+ A hypnotherapist
+ A PSYCH-K instructor
+ A naturopathic doctor
+ A nutrition specialist
+ And others, too

I especially recommend getting a chiropractor on your team. Chiropractors are somewhat overlooked and often misunderstood. Many people think that chiropractors are people who align your back after you've had an injury, like a car accident. But that's just the tip of the iceberg. Chiropractors work to align the spine, which has innumerable benefits—including boosting your immune system, and improving neural communication between your brain and the rest of your body.

When I was a teenager, I walked my dog in the woods every day. Often, I'd run into an older gentleman who walked his dog at the same time. We often chatted about nature, pets, life, and his health.

This man had faced a significant health issue when he was a child. Even back then, I was fascinated by the human body and health in general, so I always wanted to hear his stories. He was from Denmark and told me his family always used a chiropractor as the first line of defense in case of illnesses and injuries. I asked him to explain more.

Once, as a very young child, this man had a terrible bout of eczema. He was hospitalized and bandaged all over his entire body. His skin was cracked, bleeding, and full of pus because the infection was terrible. He was in and out of the hospital all the time. Finally, a chiropractor said to his parents, "Please come see me. I can help."

Seeing a chiropractor for a skin issue? Seems odd. But his father was desperate and willing to try anything, so he took his son to see the chiropractor, who did a few adjustments to create better communication through his spine to his brain and back again. This reactivated his immune system. Within a few days, his body started healing. The cracks started closing. He made a complete recovery.

The chiropractor told his father, "When your son turns about twelve or thirteen and starts going through puberty, he'll probably have a large growth spurt which may cause compression on his spine. It might trigger another eczema attack." That's exactly what happened. Fortunately, they noticed it right away and went to have another chiropractic adjustment, and that one little spot of eczema cleared up. He never suffered from it again.

This story illustrates why it's so crucial to build a Whole Health Team with several people involved. Ideally, I'd recommend having two chiropractors on your team, two naturopaths, two massage therapists, and so on. That way, if you need urgent care, you'll have a better chance at booking an appointment quickly. It's likely you'll call one office and, oops, they're fully booked up this week. That's why having two or even three providers is helpful.

Lastly, I encourage you to put together your Whole Health Team List. Start a Word document and put all your team members in one place—their emails, phone numbers, websites, office addresses, everything you need. Keep this document on your computer, on your phone, and email it to your partner or spouse. Print it out twice, put it on the fridge for everybody to see, and store it in a binder, too. Make sure everybody in your family is aware of your Whole Health Team List so they know who to call in the event you need help for an acute or chronic condition.

It will probably take you twenty to thirty minutes to pull this list together, and you'll feel so organized and empowered once you do it. With this simple action, you're signaling to yourself, "I take my health seriously."

Write Your Own Prescription

In her book *Mind Over Medicine*, Dr. Lissa Rankin urges her readers to write their own prescription for optimal health. Everyone's ideal prescription will be slightly different. What is yours?

This is a powerful exercise to do.

Get a pen and paper and ask yourself:

What Do I Need In Order to Achieve Optimal Health?

Write down everything that comes to mind. You might start with the obvious stuff, the basics. You need to eat real food. You need to get plenty of rest. You need to exercise and move your body in a way that feels energizing, not damaging. You need clean, pure, filtered water. You need a positive mindset. You need a Whole Health Team with several people working together to help you be well. You need to be a savvy, informed patient, not a passive bystander. OK, great. But what else?

When Rankin does this exercise with her patients, they often come up with creative, interesting, and sometimes surprising and emotional answers. She's had patients say:

"I need to leave my marriage." "I need to come out of the closet." "I need to quit my job." "I need to sell my house and spend some time traveling the world."

Deep down, in the clearest, brightest part of your heart, you know exactly what you need in order to thrive. You know what you need to do.

Right here, write down your personal prescription for optimal health. Write down everything you need. Keep writing for as long as you need to. It's OK if you write ten, twenty, fifty, even a hundred things. Keep going. Pour it all out.

_____

_____

_____

_____

_____

_____

_____

_____

_____

_____

_____

_____

_____

_____

_____

_____

_____

_____

_____

_____

_____

_____

_____

_____

_____

_____

_____

_____

_____

_____

_____

_____

_____

_____

_____

_____

_____

_____

I'm an optimist—but also a realist. If you just wrote down a hundred things that you need, maybe it's not feasible to have all one hundred right this instant. But I'm confident that you can have at least three of them. And then three more. And then three more.

Today, choose three items from your prescription— whichever three you can realistically bring into your life immediately. Do it. And next week, or next month, add a few more. Before long, everything you've written on your prescription pad will be...your new life.

> *"The best time to plant a tree was twenty years ago.*
> *The second-best time is now."*
>
> *—Chinese Proverb*

I love this quote so much, and it applies to every aspect of our lives. The best time to take charge of your health was five, ten, twenty years ago, or more. But today is an excellent time, too. You know exactly what kind of "tree" you need to plant and nourish. I hope you'll plant that first seed today.

A few moments ago, you created your own personal prescription for optimal health. Re-write your prescription neatly, or type it and print it out. Sign it. Make it official. Then make it happen. Your body will be so grateful, and you'll see innumerable benefits.

Whatever you want—whether it's a slimmer waistline, freedom from acne, tons of energy to write, run your business, and have fun adventures with loved ones, or a stronger chance of beating cancer so you can watch your grandkids make sand castles at the beach—whatever you want most, you have a great deal of power, and you can influence what happens next.

Will you continue onward just as you have in the past, or will you make some changes? Will you give your body every possible advantage? Will you treat your body with the utmost care and respect? Will you be the leader of your life story, or a passive bystander?

The choice is yours to make.

NEXT STEPS

Our path forward is both clear and challenging. We're embarking on a journey that involves small yet significant steps, delving into focused studies and meticulously documenting case studies. By doing so, we're not just validating our work within the academic and medical spheres, but we're also building a foundation of credibility that will be pivotal in our broader mission. These small-scale studies act as the seeds from which larger, more comprehensive research initiatives will grow. As we rigorously analyze these cases, we're equipping ourselves with the knowledge and evidence necessary to pave the way for substantial change. It's through this methodical approach that we will eventually be able to generalize our findings, affecting not just a handful of individuals, but entire communities and populations. With every case study published, we move closer to the transformative impact we aim to achieve, fostering a future where health and nutrition are accessible rights, not just for the privileged few, but for all.

No Labels

In our pursuit of optimal health, we are called upon to transcend the conventional approach of meticulously deciphering labels. The shift we need is towards consuming food that doesn't come with labels, a movement rooted in both simplicity and science.

5. The Complexity of Packaged Foods: Packaged and processed foods, adorned with intricate labels, often hide a multitude of additives, preservatives, and artificial components. These substances, designed to enhance taste and prolong shelf life, can wreak havoc on our bodies. Artificial flavors, colors, and preservatives, when ingested consistently, have been

linked to various health concerns including allergies, hyperactivity, and even carcinogenic risks.

6. Nutritional Depletion through Processing: Processing strips foods of their natural nutrients. High heat, refining, and preserving processes rob ingredients of essential vitamins, minerals, and antioxidants. The result? A product that might taste good but is nutritionally deficient. Consuming such foods consistently can lead to deficiencies and weaken our immune systems, making us more susceptible to illnesses.

7. Hidden Culprits: Labels often camouflage the presence of harmful elements like high-fructose corn syrup, excessive sodium, and unhealthy trans fats. These elements, abundant in processed foods, are notorious for contributing to diabetes, cardiovascular diseases, and obesity. The overconsumption of these substances, disguised behind the fine print, perpetuates a cycle of poor health.

8. The Whole Food Advantage: In contrast, whole, unprocessed foods offer a myriad of health benefits. Fresh fruits, vegetables, whole grains, lean proteins, and natural fats are nutrient powerhouses. They provide essential vitamins, minerals, fiber, and antioxidants vital for bodily functions. Whole foods fuel our bodies, boost our immune systems, and support overall well-being.

9. Embracing Nutrient-Rich Choices: By transitioning away from packaged foods, we embrace a lifestyle anchored in nutrient-rich, unprocessed choices. These foods, free from labels and untouched by manufacturing processes, nourish us at the cellular level. The abundance of vitamins, minerals, and antioxidants in whole foods fortifies our defenses, promoting longevity and vitality.

In our collective pursuit of lasting health, let us liberate ourselves from the confounding world of labels. Instead, let's focus on the purity and wholesomeness of foods without labels, understanding that these choices empower us, heal us, and pave the way for a healthier, vibrant tomorrow.

Higher Calling: Embracing a New Path

Our journey toward healing is guided by a force beyond us, whether you call it Pachamama, creator, God, or any other name reflecting your higher power. This universal force beckons us to embrace a transformative way of living. If we continue down our current path—filled with harmful foods and self-inflicted poisons—we will only perpetuate our suffering. The time has come for change.

During my eye-opening trip to Africa in 2019, I realized the urgent need to decolonize our diets. It struck me that many remained unaware of the historical impact of colonization, not just in our local communities but across the globe. A new paradigm is emerging, one that nurtures our bodies, minds, and puts an end to the mental health crisis and the deadly grip of chronic diseases plaguing our loved ones.

This book serves as a key to unlock this transformative journey. Open your heart as you read, but remember, the real magic transpires when you act. You possess the incredible power to reverse your chronic illness, and it starts today. I am here to support you at every step.

By joining our Eat Real to Heal six-week program, an extension of the foundational concepts presented in this book, you gain exclusive access to comprehensive guidance. Weekly group coaching sessions offer a platform to voice your questions, find inspiration from others on a similar healing path, and stay informed with the latest literature and resources. In the bewildering realm of nutrition, we are your beacon, ensuring you have access to the most up-to-date and accurate information. Together, let's embark on this healing journey and embrace the transformative power of change.

It's Your Turn to Lead

In our world starving for true healing, we urgently need pioneers—nutrition and detox experts well-versed in chronic disease reversal. The days of specialized practitioners focusing solely on one aspect of health are over. We require coaches with a holistic understanding, professionals trained comprehensively in the intricate art of total body rejuvenation. The belief that healing one part of the body in isolation suffices has proven futile; our approach must encompass all parts simultaneously.

Become a Nutrition & Detox Coach

Whether you are a seasoned healthcare practitioner, a dedicated physician, nurse, nurse practitioner, naturopath, physiotherapist, stay-at-home parent, or anyone with the desire to master the science and art of chronic disease reversal, our doors are open to you. Explore our transformative six-month program, designed not only to equip you with metabolic nutrition and detox certification but also to elevate your expertise through our Business Accelerator Program. This unique initiative empowers you to scale your existing business or launch a new venture, guiding you from ground zero to a six-figure success story within just twelve months.

Calling All BIPOC Coaches

Furthermore, if you belong to marginalized communities— Black, Indigenous, a person of color, a veteran, a single parent, or someone battling a chronic illness—we stand committed to your empowerment. Email us at info@richerhealth.ca to apply for our scholarship program. We offer a $2,000 scholarship to bridge persisting gaps in health and equity disparities, particularly affecting Black, Indigenous, and people of color. Join us in the transformative journey of healing, where your passion meets purpose, and together, we redefine the landscape of healthcare.

Going beyond Veganism and Vegetarianism

Embracing a Nutritarian and Detox Lifestyle

The culinary landscape is shifting, and we are all part of this uprising. Chefs are revolutionizing restaurants, introducing an array of vegan and plant-based options that cater to diverse tastes. Yet, amid this transformation, it's crucial to recognize that the answer lies not just in vegan or vegetarian diets but in the profound shift toward a nutritarian and detox lifestyle.

Our journey transcends the limitations of traditional veganism and vegetarianism. It delves deeper into the heart of nutrition, emphasizing a holistic approach that nourishes both body and soul. The foundation of this lifestyle rests on plant-based, whole foods—unprocessed, vibrant, and bursting with flavors that awaken your palate and leave you craving more.

Every day, you'll embark on a culinary adventure, savoring meals that are not only nutritious but also utterly delectable. It's not merely about what you eat; it's about embracing a way of life that celebrates the art of cooking, the joy of savoring every bite, and the profound impact it has on your overall well-being.

Join us in this culinary revolution, where plant-based living transcends boundaries and becomes a source of delight and fulfillment. Together, let's revel in the richness of unprocessed, whole foods, and discover the true essence of a nutritarian and detox lifestyle—one that nourishes your body, delights your senses, and elevates your life to new heights of health and happiness.

Breaking the Mold of Conventional Treatment

Understand this: what we offer is not a one-size-fits-all remedy. We're not here to apply a band-aid to your symptoms like a doctor prescribing painkillers, NSAIDs for arthritis, statins for heart issues, or IVF for infertility. We're delving deeper, addressing the very roots of your condition.

We're not just treating diseases; we're repairing your damaged tissue syndrome, revitalizing your sodium-potassium pump, eliminating insulin resistance, rejuvenating your microbiome, multiplying your mitochondria, extending your telomeres, and healing every permeable membrane in your body. We're also unblocking your micro and macro capillaries, arteries and veins, unblocking your detoxification pathways, and treating every single organ in your body at once—the list is extensive.

In our approach, we understand a fundamental truth: you can't heal one part of your body without healing everything simultaneously. This comprehensive healing method leads to a remarkable outcome: your symptoms dissolve, leaving your doctors astounded, uttering words like, "You don't need your medications anymore. Your chronic disease has vanished."

However, if your case is rare, unusual, or potentially genetic, don't hesitate to reach out. We might be able to assist, but only with the support of your entire medical team and after rigorous research. We also ask for your willingness to share your journey by allowing us to publish a case study in a peer-reviewed medical journal. Your progress can illuminate the path for others. If you're ready to explore this transformative journey, start by filling out our research application https://www.eatrealtoheal.ca/health-intake-form. Together, we can redefine what's possible in your health journey.

Summary: The Essence of the Eat Real to Heal Program

In essence, the Eat Real to Heal program is not about complicating your life; it's about simplifying and embracing a vibrant, healthful way of living. At its core, this program encourages you to turn to organic, nutrient-dense, plant-based whole foods—abundant in variety, locally sourced, and affordable. It's not about elimination; rather, it's a celebration of the incredible array of 350,000 edible plant species our planet offers.

In addition to these wholesome foods, you'll complement your diet with organic, cold-pressed vegetable juices, prepared following three specific recipes. These juices infuse your body with essential nutrients, supplementing your natural intake. To address potential deficiencies, you'll incorporate nine key pharmaceutical-grade supplements, meticulously curated to be filler and dye-free.

Moreover, the program integrates a daily liver detox, crucial for supporting your liver and kidneys in healing and detoxifying. These components—wholesome foods, nourishing juices, targeted supplements, and daily detox—are the pillars of the Eat Real to Heal program. Together, they trigger profound cellular regeneration, unblocking your body's detoxification channels. This powerful combination empowers you to combat and eliminate chronic diseases at their core.

Having worked closely with thousands of clients worldwide for nearly two decades, I stand firmly behind the effectiveness of this program. If you diligently apply the methods outlined in this book, preparing the meals, consuming the juices, taking the supplements, and adhering to the detox routines, and still find the program ineffective, I am committed to refunding your investment. My ultimate objective is to guide you toward optimal health and vitality, enabling you to unlock your true potential.

By attaining this vitality, you'll be imbued with the energy to serve others. It is through these acts of service that our communities heal, our planet thrives, and we collectively achieve true health freedom. Your journey toward optimal well-being starts here, with the simplicity and vitality of the Eat Real to Heal program.

More Resources than Ever Before

Discover a wealth of additional resources in the updated section of the book under Resources. We've curated an extensive list of books, documentaries, expert interviews, and research studies to enhance your knowledge. As the field of health and wellness continually evolves, we're dedicated to staying current. Explore this section regularly, as we frequently add new materials. For the latest updates, visit the resources page on our website www.richerhealth. ca where we ensure you have access to the most recent and relevant information each month. Knowledge is power, and we're here to empower you on your healing journey.

Empowered for Change:
Your Journey Starts Now

Congratulations! You've embarked on a transformative journey, understanding the immense power within you. You've realized that your body has incredible healing potential and that it thrives on daily hyper-nutrification and detoxification. The choices you make in every meal either build your health or compromise it—you hold the reins.

You've embraced the vital truth that your healing journey

is deeply intertwined with addressing intergenerational trauma. If you find yourself needing additional support in this area, please don't hesitate to reach out. I can connect you with therapists skilled in Internal Family Systems (IFS), Somatic Experience, and harm reduction, all rooted in trauma-informed care.

Remember, movement, sunshine, breath work, meditation, and quality sleep are essential components of your well-being. However, most clients find the latter challenging until they've restored their nutritional deficiencies and detoxified their bodies. Your body's potential for vitality is within reach.

Tips to Guide You

So, armed with this knowledge, what's your next step? Here are some tips to guide you:

1. Get a Partner: Don't tread this path alone. Having a supportive partner enhances your journey.

2. Join our Eat Real to Heal Program: Enroll in our program for ongoing support, including free weekly group coaching. Continual guidance ensures your success and prevents roadblocks.

3. Get Baseline Blood Work: Understand your starting point and track your progress. Regular blood work provides valuable insights into your health transformation.

4. Assemble Your Whole Health Team: Download our PDF guide to create a comprehensive support network. Having the right team significantly boosts your healing journey.

5. Book a Call with our Certified Coaches: Address any lingering questions or concerns with our experienced

coaches. They are here to assist you every step of the way.

6. Take the Leap: Whether it's a small step or a giant leap, start now. Your incredible life, filled with vibrant health and vitality, awaits your courageous decision.

Remember, you possess the power to shape your destiny. Your journey to optimal health starts today. Embrace it, cherish it, and witness the extraordinary transformation within you. Your future self will thank you for this momentous choice. Onward to your amazing life!

Stay Connected: Reach Out to Us!

We are here to support you every step of the way. If you have questions, need guidance, or simply want to share your progress, don't hesitate to reach out. Your journey is our priority, and we are dedicated to your success.

1. Email Us: Drop us a line at nicolette@richerhealth. ca. We're here to respond promptly and provide the assistance you need.

2. Visit Our Website: Explore our comprehensive resources, programs, and success stories at www. richerhealth.ca. Our website is a hub of valuable information designed to empower you on your path to vibrant health and well-being.

Remember, you are never alone in this journey. Your success matters to us, and we are committed to helping you achieve your health goals. Reach out, connect, and let's continue this transformative journey together.

CLOSING WORDS

You Are Not Powerless

I'm writing this book in 2017. It's been a chaotic, deeply troubling year.

North America is still reeling from the recent mass shooting in Las Vegas—an incident that claimed hundreds of lives. Our friends in Puerto Rico are living without power and shelter due to a massive hurricane. Here in Canada, we're dealing with our own wave of tragedies, including the tragic opioid epidemic. Canadians are using—and abusing—prescription painkillers like never before, leading to overdoses and death.

Our world is far from perfect. There are so many problems. Every single day, yet another crisis explodes onto the front page of the newspaper.

Many days, I hold my daughters close and I wonder, "What kind of world are they growing into? What will the future hold?" It's scary. And it's easy to feel defeated and powerless.

But the truth is, we are *not* powerless. I have a great deal of power. So do you. The power to change your eating habits. The power to change your daily routine. The power to decide what will be included in your life, and what's not permitted anymore. The power to create a new, healthier future for yourself and your family.

When It Comes to Your Health, You Are Not Powerless

You are in charge. You are the boss. You determine what your meal will be, what you'll prepare for dinner tomorrow, and what your children will have for breakfast next week. You determine whether you'll follow the guidelines in this book, or not. You choose. Because you are the author of your story, not a passive bystander.

No, you don't have the power to change everything in the entire world, but you have the power to change certain things. Many things. Starting with the way you take care of your own body.

I've stated this so many times in this book, but it bears repeating:

You Hold So Much Power

Never forget this.

Claim your power and channel this power into positive habits, nutritious meals, and a lifestyle that allows you to thrive.

I've worked with hundreds of clients in a one-on-one capacity, and I've served thousands of customers over the years through my retreats, programs, and restaurants. They've done it. They've upgraded their lifestyles. So can you. There's no doubt in my mind—you can do it, too.

I am sending love and strength to you and wishing you the best of health.

Nicolette

ACKNOWLEDGMENTS

"We, today, stand on the shoulders of our predecessors who have gone before us. We, as their successors, must catch the torch of freedom and liberty passed on to us by our ancestors. We cannot lose in this battle."

—Benjamin E. Mays

It takes a village to create a book like this one. So many people have influenced my work over the years, and so many people have supported me with their time, energy, resources, and encouragement. I stand on the shoulders of the gentle and mighty giants before me.

I thank with love and gratitude...

William Nasby for introducing me to the Gerson Therapy. Dr. Max Gerson for his persistence in bringing the Gerson Therapy to light. Charlotte Gerson and her two children, Howard and Margaret Straus, for diligently keeping the Gerson Therapy in the light, and for encouraging me to shine my light brighter too. Alexandra Franzen for her creative writing genius and for connecting me to Brenda. Stephie Hennekam for her positive vibes, attention to detail and for keeping me and this book on track. Becky Delziel and Tracy Vaughan for bringing the original *Eat Real to Heal* online course live for the world to access, learn and heal. Jaden for being my medical muse. Hazelle and Sadie for your unconditional love. My darling husband, Pierre, for going with the flow and believing in all I do and desire. Kelly Hand for spiraling me towards unapologetic greatness. Paula Jeffers for being an angel and making miracles and dreams happen—the Richer Health Retreat Centre is because of you. Erica Nasby for all the years of sharing, learning, experimenting, and uncovering the path to optimal health, wisdom, and love. Melissa Darou, you are a writing and gardening partner in crime. Marie-Lynn Tremblay for taking the leap with us and for your joyous smile that shines bright each day in our garden and wellness centre. My parents for saying yes to my vision for the Green Moustache and to all of our incredible Green Mo' staff for keeping it real so our communities can heal. Your daily presence offered up the space for this book to come to fruition. My three brothers for challenging me intellectually, supporting me with your artistic talents, humor, and for your sheer collective strength. Hayley Ingman for standing strong, true, and brave each day and for choosing us. Rachel Carson for writing *Silent Spring* and for all it has brought me ever since. Brené Brown for her tiny words of wisdom—"books can be spoken." Elizabeth Gilbert and Natalie Goldberg for *Big Magic* and *Wild Mind*. Extra love goes out to Brenda and the entire team at Mango Publishing—thank you for believing in this book, giving it a home, and ultimately for your patience as I learned to navigate this exciting world of writing and publishing. To all my clients, everywhere, who are taking their health into their own hands, returning to Food as Medicine, and working to make our planet a better place despite all the adversity you face each day. You know who you are. Bountiful Blessings.

RESOURCES

Foods to Avoid, Foods to Eat, Foods to Moderate

Foods to Avoid

+ Alcohol
+ Avocados
+ Baking soda
+ Black tea and non-herbal teas
+ Bottled or canned
+ Cheese
+ Chocolate
+ Coconut
+ Coffee
+ Dairy
+ Dehydrated or frozen
+ GMOs

+ Meat
+ Mushrooms
+ Non-organic
+ Nuts and seeds
+ Oils and fats (flaxseed oil is ok)
+ Packaged
+ Processed
+ White processed flours
+ Raw kale and raw spinach
+ Salt and salt substitutes
+ Soy

Foods to Eat In Abundance

Eat these foods morning, noon, and night. Always organic.

All organic vegetables, fruits, grains, and legumes not on the Foods To Avoid list

+ Raw fruits and veggies
+ Cooked fruits and veggies
+ Potatoes; all varieties

+ (All produce are allowed except mushrooms, avocados, the leaves of carrots and radishes, raw spinach, and mustard greens)

Foods to Eat Occasionally

I.e., once per week and only in addition to the list of foods to eat in abundance.

+ Brown rice
+ Quinoa
+ Potato flour
+ Barley

+ Lentils
+ Yams and sweet potatoes
+ Corn

Staple Pantry Items

+ Apple cider vinegar
+ Balsamic vinegar
+ Brown rice (if allowed)
+ Coffee (enemas only)
+ Distilled & filtered water
+ Flax oil (organic, not high-lignin)
+ Garlic
+ Ginger (minimal)

+ Honey
+ Maple syrup
+ Molasses (unsulfured)
+ Oatmeal
+ Onions
+ Potatoes
+ Rye bread (unsalted, non-fat, homemade)
+ Wine vinegar

Immune-Boosting Spices

Eat these in moderation, as some of the aromatic oils can slow down healing in certain people.

+ Allspice
+ Anise
+ Bay leaves
+ Chives
+ Cilantro
+ Coriander
+ Dill

+ Fennel
+ Mace
+ Marjoram
+ Parsley
+ Rosemary
+ Sage
+ Saffron

+ Scallions
+ Tarragon
+ Thyme
+ Sorrel
+ Summer savory

Example Daily Food Guide

Breakfast

+ Oatmeal and stewed fruit
+ Citrus Juice
+ Green Juice

Snacks: raw and cooked Gerson-approved foods

Lunch

+ Abundant Salad with dressing
+ 1 Cup Hippocrates Soup
+ Baked dish (three or four veggies: i.e. beets, squash, carrots)
+ Long and Low-Cooked Dish (three or four veggies: i.e. onions, tomatoes, squash, green beans)
+ Small Baked Potato
+ Carrot/Apple Juice

Snacks: raw and cooked Gerson-approved foods

Dinner

+ Abundant Salad with dressing
+ 1 Cup Hippocrates Soup
+ Baked dish (three or four veggies: i.e. beets, squash, carrots)
+ Long and Low Cooked Dish (three or four veggies: i.e. onions, tomatoes, squash, green beans)
+ Small Baked potato
+ Green Juice or Carrot/Apple Juice

Dessert examples:

+ Banana ice cream (recipe in Gerson book)
+ Apple cinnamon oat bake

Books to Read

+ *Dr. Max Gerson: Healing the Hopeless* by Howard Straus[13]

+ *A Time to Heal* by Beata Bishop

+ *Bad Science* by Ben Goldacre, MD

+ *Death by Modern Medicine* by Carolyn Dean, MD[14]

+ *Eat to Live: The Amazing Nutrient-Rich Program for Fast and Sustained Weight Loss, Revised Edition* by Joel Fuhrman

+ *Emperor of All Maladies: A Biography of Cancer* by Siddhartha Mukherjee, MD

+ *Gutbliss* by Robynne Chutkan, MD

+ *Healing the Gerson Way: Defeating Cancer and Other Chronic Diseases* by Charlotte Gerson, Beata Bishop, Joanne Shwed, Dr. Abram Hoffer

+ *How Doctors Think* by Jerome Groopman

+ *How Not to Die* by Michael Greger, MD

+ *I Contain Multitudes* by Ed Yong

+ *In Defense of Food: An Eater's Manifesto* by Michael Pollan

---

13 A must-buy! Currently, you can only buy it from here: http://store.gerson.org/Gerson-Cookbook.html or in one of our Green Moustache Cafes.
14 https://drcarolyndean.com/2014/09/death-by-modern-medicine-3rd-edition-2/

+ *Last Child in the Woods* by Richard Louv[15]

+ *Living Downstream: An Ecologist's Personal Investigation of Cancer and the Environment* by Sandra Steingraber

+ *Mind Over Medicine* by Lisa Rankin, MD[16]

+ *Nutritional Healing, After the Work of Dr. Max Gerson: A Patient Management Handbook* by Kathryn Alexander

+ *Orthomolecular Medicine for Everyone: Megavitamin Therapeutics for Families and Physicians* by Abraham Hoffer, MD, PhD, and Andrew Saul, MD, PhD

+ *Pleasure Trap: Mastering the Hidden Force that Undermines Health & Happiness* by Doug J. Lisle and Alan Goldhamer

+ *Proteinaholic* by Garth Davis, MD[17]

+ *Salt Sugar Fat: How the Food Giants Hooked Us* by Michael Moss

+ *The Alzheimer's Solution: A Breakthrough Program to Prevent and Reverse the Symptoms of Cognitive Decline at Every Age* by Dean Sherzai, MD, and Ayesha Sherzai, MD

+ *The Brain That Changes Itself: Stories of Personal Triumph from the Frontiers of Brain Science* by Norman Doidge

+ *The Gerson Therapy Cookbook*

+ *The Nature of Crops: How We Came to Eat the*

---

15 http://richardlouv.com/books/last-child/
16 http://mindovermedicinebook.com/
17 http://proteinaholic.com/

Plants We Do by J. Warren

✦ *The Other Side of Impossible* by Susannah Meadows

✦ *The Pleasure Trap* by Alan Goldhamer

✦ *The China Study* by T. Colin Campbell

✦ *Unprocessed: How to Achieve Vibrant Health and Your Ideal Weight* by Chef AJ

Documentaries to Watch

Cowspiracy

Dominion

Dying to have known

Eating Animals

Eating Our Way to Extinction

Fed Up

Food Inc.

Forks over Knives

Heal yourself, Heal the world

In Defense of Food

PlantPure Nation

Simply Raw: Reversing Diabetes in 30 Days

Speciesism

The Beautiful Truth

The Burzynski Movie

The C-Word

The Food Cure

The Game Changers

The Gerson Miracle

Vegucated

What the Health

Movies to Watch

Concussion

Erin Brockovich

Love & Other Drugs

Miracles from Heaven

The Dallas Buyers Club

Dr. Max Gerson: The Forbidden Cure (coming soon)

People to Follow

Alan Goldhamer, DC

Caldwell Esselstyn, MD

Dean Ornish, MD

Garth Davis, MD

Joel Fuhrman, MD

Joel Kahn, MD

Kim Williams, MD

Michael Greger, MD

Neal Barnard, MD

T. Colin Campbell, PhD

Valter Longo, PhD

Zach Bush, MD

Julianna Hever, MS, RD, CPT

Rich Roll Podcast

NICOLETTE RICHER

Nicolette Richer is an Orthomolecular Health Educator, Gerson Therapy Home Set-Up Trainer, and Psycho-Kinaesthetic Facilitator.

Her education includes a MA in Environmental Education and Communication, a BA in Interdisciplinary Studies, and a certificate in Sustainable Community Development. She's currently working on her Doctor of Social Sciences degree at Royal Roads University.

She's a former environmental and sustainability consultant who spent many years studying the connection between toxicity in the soil, air, and water and chronic diseases.

Today, she runs several businesses—a collection of 100 percent organic cafes called the Green Moustache, with eight locations across Canada as of today. She's been running Richer Health Consulting for over a decade, where she offers one-on-one consulting, workshops, speaking, online courses, and events. Recently, she launched the Richer Heath Retreat Center, a sanctuary in British Columbia offering transformational retreats for people battling cancer, diabetes, heart disease, fatigue, depression, and many other conditions. She's also the founder of Sea to Sky Thrivers Society, an NGO that works with youth and indigenous communities to remember the art and science of traditional whole foods as medicine.

Nicolette's mission is to empower people to take their health into their own hands, to demonstrate how food can be used as healing medicine, and to show people that leading a healthy lifestyle doesn't have to be boring—it can be colorful, inspiring, and fun.

You can find Nicolette's projects online at:

greenmoustache.com
seatoskythrivers.com
richerhealth.ca
eatrealtoheal.ca
richerhealthretreatcentre.com

ABOUT THE
GREEN MOUSTACHE

Come eat with us!

Visit the Green Moustache Organic Café and juice bar at one of our eight locations.

We'd love to show you that eating real food can be incredibly satisfying and delicious. One meal, and you'll be hooked.

Green Moustache Organic Café Locations

1. Whistler Village, BC
2. Function Junction, Whistler, BC
3. Squamish, BC
4. Edgemont Village, West Vancouver, BC
5. Lower Lonsdale, North Vancouver, BC
6. Port Moody, BC
7. Revelstoke, BC
8. Edmonton, BC

Open Your Own Location

Do you dream about running your own business?

Want to work in a fun, colorful, crunchy, creamy, zingy environment surrounded by beautiful organic food and passionate people?

Want to make a positive difference in your hometown by providing organic, plant-based meals that nutrify and detoxify people's bodies?

If you'd like information on how to open your own Green Mo' franchise location, visit: **greenmoustache.com/franchise**.

On that page, we have a quick application that you can fill out, and then we'll be in touch soon. Thank you!

Mango Publishing, established in 2014, publishes an eclectic list of books by diverse authors—both new and established voices—on topics ranging from business, personal growth, women's empowerment, LGBTQ studies, health, and spirituality to history, popular culture, time management, decluttering, lifestyle, mental wellness, aging, and sustainable living. We were named 2019 and 2020's #1 fastest growing independent publisher by Publishers Weekly. Our success is driven by our main goal, which is to publish high-quality books that will entertain readers as well as make a positive difference in their lives.

Our readers are our most important resource; we value your input, suggestions, and ideas. We'd love to hear from you—after all, we are publishing books for you!

Please stay in touch with us and follow us at:

Facebook: Mango Publishing
Twitter: @MangoPublishing
Instagram: @MangoPublishing
LinkedIn: Mango Publishing
Pinterest: Mango Publishing
Newsletter: mangopublishinggroup.com/newsletter

Join us on Mango's journey to reinvent publishing, one book at a time.